*Welcome to the **"Type 2 Diabetes Cookbook for 1 Person: 110+ Quick and Healthy Recipes for Busy Individuals with Type 2 Diabetes."** This cookbook is your essential companion to managing diabetes with delicious, nutritious meals designed specifically for solo dining.*

Living with Type 2 diabetes requires thoughtful consideration of your diet, but it shouldn't mean sacrificing flavor or spending hours in the kitchen. This book is crafted to offer a variety of quick and easy recipes that are both satisfying and supportive of blood sugar control.

Inside these pages, you'll discover over 110 recipes tailored for one person, each created to be simple to prepare without compromising on taste or nutritional value. From hearty breakfasts to satisfying lunches and comforting dinners, every dish is designed to help you maintain stable blood sugar levels while enjoying your meals.

In addition to mouth-watering recipes, this cookbook provides practical tips and guidance on portion control, ingredient substitutions, and efficient meal planning strategies. These insights are aimed at making it easier for busy individuals to integrate healthy eating habits seamlessly into their daily lives.

Whether you're newly diagnosed with Type 2 diabetes or looking for fresh, inspiring meal ideas, this book is here to support you on your journey to better health. Explore a wide range of flavors and culinary delights that prove managing diabetes can be both manageable and enjoyable.

Get ready to embark on a culinary adventure where every recipe is crafted with your health and taste buds in mind. Here's to delicious meals, stable blood sugar, and a healthier, happier you!

1. Vegetable Omelet

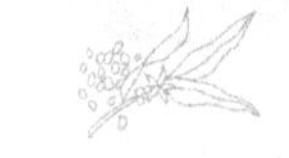

PREP TIME
20 MINUTES

COOK TIME
30 MINUTES

INGREDIENTS:

- 3 eggs
- 2 tbsp milk or water
- 1 tbsp butter or oil
- 1/4 cup diced vegetables (such as bell peppers, onions, mushrooms, spinach)
- Salt and pepper to taste
- Shredded cheese (optional)

PROCEDURE:

1. Crack the eggs into a small bowl and beat them lightly with the milk or water. Season with a pinch of salt and pepper.

2. Heat a small non-stick skillet over medium heat and melt the butter or heat the oil.

3. Pour the egg mixture into the pan and let it sit for 20-30 seconds to set the bottom.

4. Use a spatula to gently push the cooked egg towards the center, tilting the pan to allow the uncooked egg to flow to the edges.

5. When the eggs are mostly set but still a bit wet on top, add the diced vegetables evenly over the top.

6. Fold the omelet in half and slide it onto a plate.

7. Top with shredded cheese if desired.

8. Serve hot and enjoy!

You can customize the omelet by using your favorite fresh vegetables. This makes a quick, healthy, and delicious breakfast or brunch.

2. Greek Yogurt with Berries

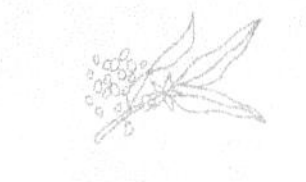

PREP TIME
20 MINUTES

COOK TIME
30 MINUTES

INGREDIENTS :

- 1 cup plain Greek yogurt (full-fat or low-fat)
- 1/2 cup fresh or frozen berries (such as blueberries, raspberries, or blackberries)
- 1 tsp honey (optional)
- Cinnamon (optional)

PROCEDURE :

1. Scoop the Greek yogurt into a bowl or serving dish.

2. Top the yogurt with the fresh or frozen berries.

3. If desired, drizzle the honey over the top of the berries.

4. Sprinkle a light dusting of cinnamon over the top (cinnamon can help regulate blood sugar levels).

That's it! This simple and delicious parfait-style dish provides several benefits for managing type 2 diabetes:

- Greek yogurt is high in protein, which helps keep you feeling full and satisfied. The protein also helps stabilize blood sugar levels.

- Berries are low in carbs and high in fiber, which also helps control blood sugar spikes.

- The healthy fats in full-fat Greek yogurt can help slow the absorption of carbs.

- Honey and cinnamon are optional, but can provide additional blood sugar-regulating benefits.

This makes a great breakfast, snack, or light dessert. Adjust the portions as needed to fit your individual dietary needs for managing type 2 diabetes.

3. Chia Seed Pudding

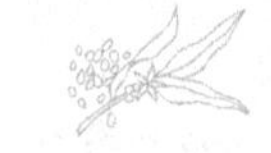

PREP TIME
20 MINUTES

COOK TIME
30 MINUTES

INGREDIENTS:

- 1/4 cup chia seeds
- 1 cup unsweetened almond milk (or other non-dairy milk)
- 1 tbsp honey or maple syrup (optional)
- 1/2 tsp vanilla extract
- Pinch of cinnamon (optional)
- Fresh berries or sliced almonds for topping (optional)

PROCEDURE:

1. In a medium bowl, whisk together the chia seeds and almond milk until well combined.

2. Stir in the honey/maple syrup (if using) and vanilla extract.

3. Cover the bowl and refrigerate for at least 2 hours, or overnight, stirring occasionally, until the mixture has thickened to a pudding-like consistency.

4. When ready to serve, give the pudding a final stir. Top with fresh berries, sliced almonds, or a sprinkle of cinnamon if desired.

This chia seed pudding is an excellent option for managing type 2 diabetes for a few reasons:

- Chia seeds are high in fiber, which helps slow the absorption of carbs and stabilize blood sugar levels.

- Chia seeds are also a good source of protein, healthy fats, and antioxidants.

- Unsweetened almond milk is low in carbs and calories compared to regular dairy milk.

- The optional honey or maple syrup provides a touch of sweetness without spiking blood sugar too much.

- Berries and cinnamon can also help regulate blood sugar.

This pudding makes a satisfying, nutrient-dense breakfast, snack or dessert. Adjust the sweetener to your taste preferences and dietary needs.

4. Avocado Toast on Whole Grain Bread

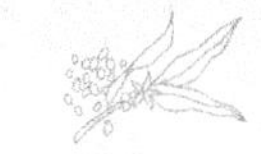

PREP TIME
20 MINUTES

COOK TIME
30 MINUTES

INGREDIENTS :

- 2 slices of whole grain or sprouted bread
- 1/2 ripe avocado, mashed
- 1 tbsp olive oil
- 1 tsp lemon juice
- Salt and pepper to taste
- Optional toppings: sliced tomatoes, sliced radishes, everything bagel seasoning, red pepper flakes

PROCEDURE :

1. Toast the whole grain bread until lightly golden brown.

2. In a small bowl, mash the avocado with the olive oil and lemon juice. Season with a pinch of salt and pepper.

3. Spread the mashed avocado evenly over the toasted bread slices.

4. Top the avocado toast with any desired additional toppings, such as sliced tomatoes, radishes, everything bagel seasoning, or red pepper flakes.

This avocado toast makes a great option for managing type 2 diabetes for a few reasons:

- Whole grain bread is high in fiber, which helps slow the absorption of carbs and stabilize blood sugar levels.

- Avocado is high in healthy monounsaturated fats, which can help improve insulin sensitivity.

- The healthy fats and fiber in avocado also help keep you feeling full and satisfied.

- Lemon juice and optional toppings like tomatoes and radishes provide additional nutrients and antioxidants.

This makes a nutritious and filling breakfast or snack. You can adjust the portion size as needed to fit your individual dietary needs for managing type 2 diabetes. Enjoy!

5. Overnight Oats with Almond Milk

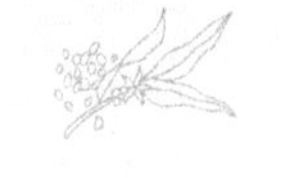

PREP TIME
20 MINUTES

COOK TIME
30 MINUTES

INGREDIENTS :

- 1/2 cup rolled oats
- 1 cup unsweetened almond milk
- 1 tbsp chia seeds
- 1 tsp honey or maple syrup (optional)
- 1/2 tsp vanilla extract
- Cinnamon to taste
- Fresh berries or sliced almonds for topping (optional)

PROCEDURE :

1. In a medium-sized bowl or mason jar, combine the rolled oats, almond milk, chia seeds, honey/maple syrup (if using), and vanilla extract. Stir well to combine.

2. Cover the bowl or seal the mason jar and refrigerate overnight, or for at least 4-6 hours.

3. When ready to serve, give the oats a good stir. Top with fresh berries, sliced almonds, and an extra sprinkle of cinnamon if desired.

This overnight oats recipe is an excellent choice for managing type 2 diabetes for several reasons:

- Rolled oats are a complex carb that is high in fiber, which helps slow the absorption of carbs and stabilize blood sugar levels.

- Unsweetened almond milk is low in carbs and calories compared to regular dairy milk.

- Chia seeds are high in fiber, protein, and healthy fats, which can also help regulate blood sugar.

- The optional honey or maple syrup provides a touch of sweetness without spiking blood sugar too much.

- Cinnamon has been shown to help improve insulin sensitivity.

- Berries and nuts add extra fiber, antioxidants, and healthy fats.

This makes a nutritious and satisfying breakfast or snack. You can adjust the sweetener and toppings to your personal taste preferences and dietary needs.

6. Scrambled Tofu with Vegetables

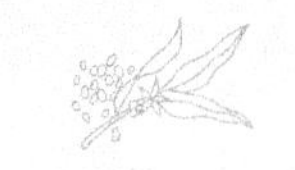

PREP TIME
20 MINUTES

COOK TIME
30 MINUTES

INGREDIENTS :

- 1 block (14 oz) firm or extra-firm tofu, crumbled
- 1 tbsp olive oil
- 1/2 cup diced onion
- 1 cup diced bell peppers
- 1 cup sliced mushrooms
- 2 cups baby spinach, chopped
- 1 tsp ground turmeric
- 1/2 tsp ground cumin
- 1/4 tsp garlic powder
- Salt and pepper to taste

PROCEDURE :

1. Heat the olive oil in a large skillet over medium heat. Add the diced onion and sauté for 2-3 minutes until translucent.

2. Add the diced bell peppers and sliced mushrooms to the skillet. Sauté for 5 minutes, stirring occasionally, until the vegetables are tender.

3. Crumble the tofu into the skillet and use a spatula to break it up into small pieces.

4. Stir in the turmeric, cumin, garlic powder, salt, and pepper. Cook for 5-7 minutes, stirring occasionally, until the tofu is heated through.

5. Add the chopped spinach and continue cooking for 2-3 minutes, until the spinach is wilted. Remove from heat and serve hot.

This scrambled tofu with vegetables is a great option for managing type 2 diabetes for several reasons:
- Tofu is high in protein and low in carbs, making it a diabetes-friendly protein source.

- The vegetables like bell peppers, mushrooms, and spinach are packed with fiber, vitamins, and minerals while being very low in carbs.

- The spices like turmeric and cumin have anti-inflammatory properties and may help improve insulin sensitivity.

- The healthy fats from the olive oil can also help regulate blood sugar levels.

This makes a satisfying and nutritious breakfast, brunch, or light meal. Adjust the seasoning and vegetable mix to your taste preferences. Enjoy!

7. Cottage Cheese with Fresh Fruit

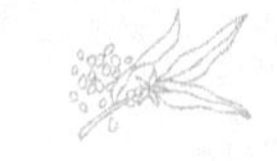

PREP TIME
20 MINUTES

COOK TIME
30 MINUTES

INGREDIENTS:

- 1 cup low-fat or non-fat cottage cheese
- 1/2 cup fresh fruit (such as berries, sliced peaches, or diced melon)
- 1 tsp honey (optional)
- Cinnamon (optional)

PROCEDURE:

1. Scoop the cottage cheese into a bowl or serving dish.

2. Top the cottage cheese with the fresh fruit of your choice.

3. If desired, drizzle the honey over the top of the fruit.

4. Sprinkle a light dusting of cinnamon over the top (cinnamon can help regulate blood sugar levels).

This cottage cheese and fresh fruit dish is a great option for managing type 2 diabetes for several reasons:

- Cottage cheese is high in protein, which helps keep you feeling full and satisfied. The protein also helps stabilize blood sugar levels.

- Fresh fruit provides fiber, vitamins, and natural sweetness without spiking blood sugar too much. Berries, in particular, are very low in carbs.

- The optional honey provides a touch of sweetness, but in moderation it won't cause a dramatic blood sugar spike.

- Cinnamon has been shown to help improve insulin sensitivity.

This makes a refreshing and nutritious breakfast, snack, or light dessert. You can adjust the portion sizes of the cottage cheese and fruit to fit your individual dietary needs for managing type 2 diabetes. Enjoy!

8. Smoothie with Spinach, Berries, and Protein Powder

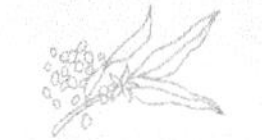 

PREP TIME
20 MINUTES

COOK TIME
30 MINUTES

INGREDIENTS :

- 1 cup unsweetened almond milk
- 1 cup fresh spinach
- 1 cup frozen mixed berries (such as blueberries, raspberries, and blackberries)
- 1 scoop unflavored or vanilla protein powder
- 1 tbsp chia seeds (optional)
- 1 tsp honey (optional)

PROCEDURE :

1. Add the almond milk, spinach, frozen berries, protein powder, and chia seeds (if using) to a high-powered blender.

2. Blend on high speed until the mixture is smooth and creamy, about 1-2 minutes.

3. If desired, drizzle in the honey and blend again briefly to incorporate.

4. Pour the smoothie into a glass and enjoy immediately.

This spinach, berry, and protein powder smoothie is a great option for managing type 2 diabetes for several reasons:

- Spinach is packed with fiber, vitamins, and minerals while being very low in carbs.

- Berries are low in carbs and high in fiber, antioxidants, and other beneficial nutrients.

- Protein powder helps provide a steady source of protein to help stabilize blood sugar levels.

- Chia seeds add extra fiber, protein, and healthy fats.

- The optional honey provides a touch of sweetness without spiking blood sugar too much.

- Unsweetened almond milk is low in carbs and calories compared to regular dairy milk.

This makes a nutritious and filling breakfast or snack. You can adjust the amounts of ingredients to suit your individual dietary needs for managing type 2 diabetes. Enjoy!

9. Quinoa Breakfast Bowl

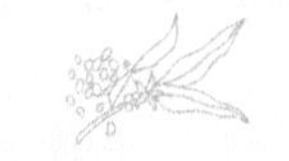

PREP TIME
20 MINUTES

COOK TIME
30 MINUTES

INGREDIENTS:

- 1/2 cup cooked quinoa, cooled
- 1/2 cup unsweetened almond milk
- 1 tbsp chia seeds
- 1 tsp honey (optional)
- 1/2 cup fresh berries (such as blueberries, raspberries, or blackberries)
- 2 tbsp sliced almonds
- Cinnamon to taste

PROCEDURE:

1. In a medium bowl, combine the cooked quinoa, almond milk, and chia seeds. Stir well.

2. If desired, drizzle the honey over the quinoa mixture and stir to incorporate.

3. Top the quinoa with the fresh berries and sliced almonds.

4. Sprinkle a light dusting of cinnamon over the top.

This quinoa breakfast bowl is a great option for managing type 2 diabetes for several reasons:

- Quinoa is a whole grain that is high in fiber, protein, and complex carbs, which can help stabilize blood sugar levels.

- Unsweetened almond milk is low in carbs and calories compared to regular dairy milk.

- Chia seeds are high in fiber, protein, and healthy fats, which can also help regulate blood sugar.

- Berries are low in carbs and high in fiber, vitamins, and antioxidants.

- Almonds provide healthy fats and a crunchy texture.

- Cinnamon has been shown to help improve insulin sensitivity.

This makes a nutritious and satisfying breakfast. You can adjust the portions of quinoa, milk, and toppings to fit your individual dietary needs for managing type 2 diabetes. Enjoy!

10. Low-Carb Pancakes

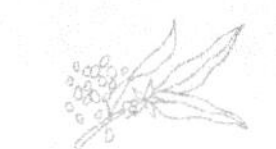

PREP TIME
20 MINUTES

COOK TIME
30 MINUTES

INGREDIENTS:

- 2 eggs
- 1/4 cup almond flour
- 1 tbsp coconut flour
- 1 tsp baking powder
- 1/4 tsp cinnamon
- 1/4 cup unsweetened almond milk
- 1 tsp vanilla extract
- 1 tbsp butter or coconut oil for cooking

Optional Toppings:
- Fresh berries
- Unsweetened shredded coconut
- Chopped nuts
- Sugar-free maple syrup

PROCEDURE:

1. In a medium bowl, whisk together the eggs, almond flour, coconut flour, baking powder, and cinnamon until well combined.

2. Stir in the almond milk and vanilla extract until a smooth batter forms.

3. Heat a non-stick skillet or griddle over medium heat and melt the butter or coconut oil.

4. Scoop the batter onto the hot surface, using about 2-3 tablespoons per pancake.

5. Cook for 2-3 minutes per side, until golden brown.

6. Serve the low-carb pancakes warm, topped with your choice of fresh berries, shredded coconut, chopped nuts, or a drizzle of sugar-free maple syrup.

These low-carb pancakes are a great option for managing type 2 diabetes for several reasons:

- Almond flour and coconut flour are low in carbs and high in fiber, which helps prevent blood sugar spikes.
- Eggs provide protein to help stabilize blood sugar levels.
- The optional toppings like berries, nuts, and sugar-free syrup add flavor without too many carbs.
- The recipe is free of refined flours and added sugars.

This makes a satisfying and diabetes-friendly breakfast. Adjust the portion sizes as needed to fit your individual dietary requirements. Enjoy!

11. Egg Muffins with Veggies

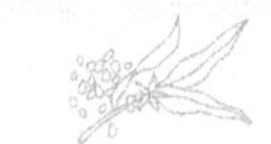 

PREP TIME
20 MINUTES

COOK TIME
30 MINUTES

INGREDIENTS :

- 8 large eggs
- 1/2 cup diced bell peppers
- 1/2 cup diced onions
- 1 cup chopped spinach or kale
- 2 tbsp grated Parmesan cheese (optional)
- Salt and pepper to taste

PROCEDURE :

1. Preheat your oven to 350°F (175°C). Grease a 12-cup muffin tin with non-stick cooking spray.

2. In a large bowl, whisk the eggs together.

3. Stir in the diced bell peppers, onions, and chopped spinach/kale. Season with salt and pepper.

4. Divide the egg mixture evenly among the 12 muffin cups.

5. If using, sprinkle the grated Parmesan cheese on top of each muffin.

6. Bake for 20-25 minutes, until the eggs are set and the tops are lightly golden.

7. Allow the egg muffins to cool for 5 minutes before removing them from the tin.

These egg muffins with veggies are a great option for managing type 2 diabetes for several reasons:

- Eggs are an excellent source of protein, which helps stabilize blood sugar levels.
- The vegetables like bell peppers, onions, and spinach/kale add fiber, vitamins, and minerals while being very low in carbs.
- The optional Parmesan cheese provides a boost of healthy fats.
- The muffin format makes them easy to grab-and-go for a quick, diabetes-friendly breakfast or snack.

You can customize the veggie mix to your liking. These egg muffins can be made ahead of time and reheated as needed throughout the week. Adjust the portion size to fit your individual dietary needs for managing type 2 diabetes.

12. Whole Grain Toast with Nut Butter

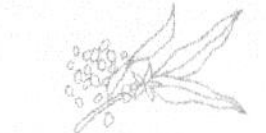 

PREP TIME
20 MINUTES

COOK TIME
30 MINUTES

INGREDIENTS :

- 2 slices of whole grain or sprouted bread
- 2 tbsp natural nut butter (such as peanut, almond, or cashew butter)
- Optional toppings: sliced banana, berries, cinnamon, chia seeds

PROCEDURE :

1. Toast the whole grain or sprouted bread until lightly golden brown.

2. Spread 1 tbsp of the natural nut butter evenly over each slice of toast.

3. Top the nut butter toast with any desired toppings, such as sliced banana, fresh berries, a sprinkle of cinnamon, or a sprinkle of chia seeds.

This whole grain toast with nut butter makes a great option for managing type 2 diabetes for a few reasons:

- Whole grain bread is high in fiber, which helps slow the absorption of carbs and stabilize blood sugar levels.

- Natural nut butters are a good source of healthy fats and protein, which can also help regulate blood sugar.

- The fiber, protein, and healthy fats in this snack help keep you feeling full and satisfied.

- Optional toppings like banana, berries, and cinnamon provide additional nutrients and antioxidants that can further help manage diabetes.

This makes a quick and easy breakfast, snack, or light meal. You can adjust the portion size of the nut butter and toppings to fit your individual dietary needs for managing type 2 diabetes. Enjoy!

13. Berry and Spinach Smoothie

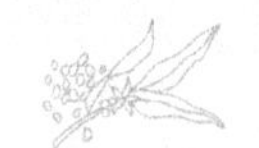

PREP TIME
20 MINUTES

COOK TIME
30 MINUTES

INGREDIENTS:

- 1 cup unsweetened almond milk
- 1 cup fresh spinach
- 1 cup frozen mixed berries (such as blueberries, raspberries, and blackberries)
- 1 tbsp chia seeds
- 1 tbsp almond butter (optional)
- 1 tsp honey (optional)

PROCEDURE:

1. Add all the ingredients to a high-powered blender.

2. Blend on high speed until the mixture is smooth and creamy, about 1-2 minutes.

3. Pour the smoothie into a glass and enjoy immediately.

This berry and spinach smoothie is an excellent choice for managing type 2 diabetes for several reasons:

- Spinach is packed with fiber, vitamins, and minerals while being very low in carbs.

- Berries are low in carbs and high in fiber, antioxidants, and other beneficial nutrients.

- Chia seeds add extra fiber, protein, and healthy fats to help regulate blood sugar.

- Almond butter provides healthy fats and a creamy texture.

- The optional honey provides a touch of sweetness without spiking blood sugar too much.

- Unsweetened almond milk is low in carbs and calories compared to regular dairy milk.

This makes a nutritious and filling breakfast or snack. You can adjust the amounts of ingredients to suit your individual dietary needs for managing type 2 diabetes. Enjoy!

14. Buckwheat Pancakes

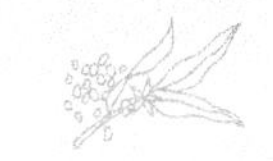

PREP TIME
20 MINUTES

COOK TIME
30 MINUTES

INGREDIENTS :

- 1 cup buckwheat flour
- 1 tsp baking powder
- 1/4 tsp salt
- 1 egg
- 1 cup unsweetened almond milk
- 1 tbsp melted coconut oil or butter
- 1 tsp vanilla extract
- Optional toppings: fresh berries, sliced almonds, unsweetened shredded coconut, sugar-free maple syrup

PROCEDURE :

1. In a medium bowl, whisk together the buckwheat flour, baking powder, and salt.

2. In a separate bowl, beat the egg. Then stir in the almond milk, melted coconut oil/butter, and vanilla extract.

3. Pour the wet ingredients into the dry ingredients and stir just until combined (do not overmix).

4. Heat a non-stick skillet or griddle over medium heat. Lightly grease the surface with additional coconut oil or butter if needed.

5. Scoop about 1/4 cup of the batter onto the hot surface for each pancake. Cook for 2-3 minutes per side, until golden brown.

6. Serve the buckwheat pancakes warm, topped with your choice of fresh berries, sliced almonds, unsweetened shredded coconut, and/or a drizzle of sugar-free maple syrup.

These buckwheat pancakes are a great option for managing type 2 diabetes for several reasons:

- Buckwheat flour is a gluten-free, low-glycemic grain that is high in fiber and protein, helping to stabilize blood sugar levels.
- Almond milk is low in carbs and calories compared to regular dairy milk.
- Eggs provide protein to help keep you feeling full.
- The optional toppings like berries, nuts, and sugar-free syrup add flavor without too many carbs.

This makes a satisfying and diabetes-friendly breakfast. Adjust the portion sizes as needed to fit your individual dietary requirements. Enjoy!

15. Oatmeal with Nuts and Berries

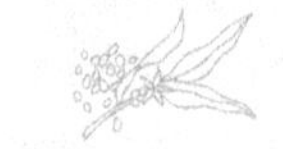 

PREP TIME
20 MINUTES

COOK TIME
30 MINUTES

INGREDIENTS :

- 1/2 cup rolled oats
- 1 cup unsweetened almond milk (or other non-dairy milk)
- 1 tbsp chopped walnuts or almonds
- 1/2 cup fresh or frozen berries (such as blueberries, raspberries, or blackberries)
- 1 tsp cinnamon
- 1 tsp honey (optional)

PROCEDURE :

1. In a small saucepan, combine the rolled oats and almond milk. Bring to a simmer over medium heat.

2. Reduce heat to low and cook the oatmeal, stirring occasionally, for 5-7 minutes until thickened to your desired consistency.

3. Remove the oatmeal from heat and stir in the chopped nuts, berries, and cinnamon.

4. If desired, drizzle the honey over the top of the oatmeal.

This oatmeal with nuts and berries is an excellent choice for managing type 2 diabetes for several reasons:

- Rolled oats are a complex carb that is high in fiber, which helps slow the absorption of carbs and stabilize blood sugar levels.

- Nuts like walnuts and almonds provide healthy fats and protein to help keep you feeling full and satisfied.

- Berries are low in carbs and high in fiber, vitamins, and antioxidants.

- Cinnamon has been shown to help improve insulin sensitivity.

- The optional honey provides a touch of sweetness without spiking blood sugar too much.

This makes a nutritious and filling breakfast. You can adjust the portions of oats, nuts, and berries to fit your individual dietary needs for managing type 2 diabetes. Enjoy!

16. Tofu Scramble with Spinach

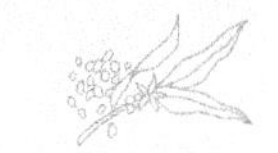

PREP TIME
20 MINUTES

COOK TIME
30 MINUTES

INGREDIENTS :

- 1 block (14 oz) firm or extra-firm tofu, crumbled
- 1 tbsp olive oil
- 1/2 cup diced onion
- 2 cloves garlic, minced
- 1 cup fresh spinach, chopped
- 1 tsp ground turmeric
- 1/2 tsp ground cumin
- 1/4 tsp garlic powder
- Salt and pepper to taste
- Optional toppings: sliced avocado, salsa, hot sauce

PROCEDURE :

1. Heat the olive oil in a large skillet over medium heat. Add the diced onion and sauté for 2-3 minutes until translucent.

2. Add the minced garlic and sauté for another 1 minute until fragrant.

3. Crumble the tofu into the skillet and use a spatula to break it up into small pieces.

4. Stir in the turmeric, cumin, garlic powder, salt, and pepper. Cook for 5-7 minutes, stirring occasionally, until the tofu is heated through.

5. Add the chopped spinach and continue cooking for 2-3 minutes, until the spinach is wilted.

6. Remove from heat and serve hot, optionally topped with sliced avocado, salsa, or hot sauce.

This tofu scramble is a great option for managing type 2 diabetes for several reasons:

- Tofu is high in protein and low in carbs, making it a diabetes-friendly protein source.

- Spinach is packed with fiber, vitamins, and minerals while being very low in carbs.

- The spices like turmeric and cumin have anti-inflammatory properties and may help improve insulin sensitivity.

- Healthy fats from the olive oil and optional avocado topping can also help regulate blood sugar levels.

This makes a satisfying and nutritious breakfast or brunch. Adjust the seasoning and toppings to your taste preferences. Enjoy!

17. Cottage Cheese and Pineapple

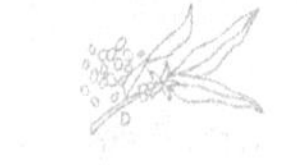 

PREP TIME
20 MINUTES

COOK TIME
30 MINUTES

INGREDIENTS:

- 1 cup low-fat or non-fat cottage cheese
- 1/2 cup fresh pineapple chunks
- 1 tsp honey (optional)
- Cinnamon (optional)

PROCEDURE:

1. Scoop the cottage cheese into a bowl or serving dish.

2. Top the cottage cheese with the fresh pineapple chunks.

3. If desired, drizzle the honey over the top of the pineapple.

4. Sprinkle a light dusting of cinnamon over the top (cinnamon can help regulate blood sugar levels).

This cottage cheese and pineapple dish is a great option for managing type 2 diabetes for several reasons:

- Cottage cheese is high in protein, which helps keep you feeling full and satisfied. The protein also helps stabilize blood sugar levels.

- Pineapple provides natural sweetness and fiber, without spiking blood sugar too much. Pineapple is also a good source of vitamin C.

- The optional honey provides a touch of sweetness, but in moderation it won't cause a dramatic blood sugar spike.

- Cinnamon has been shown to help improve insulin sensitivity.

This makes a refreshing and nutritious snack or light breakfast. You can adjust the portion sizes of the cottage cheese and pineapple to fit your individual dietary needs for managing type 2 diabetes. Enjoy!

18. Breakfast Burrito with Veggies

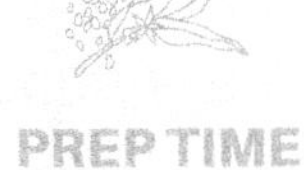 

PREP TIME
20 MINUTES

COOK TIME
30 MINUTES

INGREDIENTS :

- 2 eggs, scrambled
- 1/4 cup diced bell peppers
- 1/4 cup diced onions
- 1/2 cup baby spinach, chopped
- 2 tbsp shredded cheddar cheese
- 1 whole wheat or low-carb tortilla
- Salt and pepper to taste

PROCEDURE :

1. In a non-stick skillet, scramble the eggs over medium heat until cooked through. Season with a pinch of salt and pepper.

2. Add the diced bell peppers and onions to the skillet. Sauté for 2-3 minutes until the vegetables are tender.

3. Stir in the chopped spinach and cook for another 1-2 minutes until the spinach is wilted.

4. Remove the vegetable-egg mixture from heat and stir in the shredded cheddar cheese.

5. Lay the tortilla flat on a plate or work surface. Spoon the cheesy vegetable-egg mixture onto the center of the tortilla.

6. Fold the bottom of the tortilla up over the filling, then fold in the sides and continue rolling up into a burrito shape. Serve the breakfast burrito warm.

This breakfast burrito with veggies is a great option for managing type 2 diabetes for several reasons:

- Eggs provide protein to help stabilize blood sugar levels.
- The vegetables like bell peppers, onions, and spinach add fiber, vitamins, and minerals while being very low in carbs.
- Whole wheat or low-carb tortillas are a better choice than refined flour tortillas.
- The small amount of cheddar cheese provides healthy fats without too many carbs.

This makes a satisfying and nutritious breakfast. You can adjust the vegetable fillings to your preferences. Enjoy!

19. Protein-Packed Smoothie

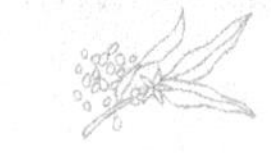

PREP TIME
20 MINUTES

COOK TIME
30 MINUTES

INGREDIENTS :

- 1 cup unsweetened almond milk
- 1/2 cup plain Greek yogurt
- 1 scoop unflavored or vanilla protein powder
- 1/2 cup frozen mixed berries
- 1 tbsp almond butter
- 1 tbsp chia seeds
- 1 tsp honey (optional)

PROCEDURE :

1. Add all the ingredients to a high-powered blender.

2. Blend on high speed until the mixture is smooth and creamy, about 1-2 minutes.

3. Pour the smoothie into a glass and enjoy immediately.

This protein-packed smoothie is an excellent choice for managing type 2 diabetes for several reasons:

- Greek yogurt is high in protein, which helps stabilize blood sugar levels.

- Protein powder provides an additional boost of protein to keep you feeling full and satisfied.

- Berries are low in carbs and high in fiber, vitamins, and antioxidants.

- Almond butter adds healthy fats and a creamy texture.

- Chia seeds contribute fiber, protein, and healthy omega-3s.

- The optional honey provides a touch of sweetness without spiking blood sugar too much.

- Unsweetened almond milk is low in carbs and calories compared to regular dairy milk.

This makes a nutritious and filling breakfast or snack. You can adjust the amounts of ingredients to suit your individual dietary needs for managing type 2 diabetes. Enjoy!

20. Whole Grain English Muffin with Avocado

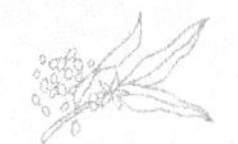

PREP TIME
20 MINUTES

COOK TIME
30 MINUTES

INGREDIENTS :

- 1 whole grain English muffin, toasted
- 1/2 ripe avocado, mashed
- 1 tsp olive oil
- 1 tsp lemon juice
- Salt and pepper to taste
- Optional toppings: sliced tomatoes, everything bagel seasoning, red pepper flakes

PROCEDURE :

1. Toast the whole grain English muffin until lightly golden brown.

2. In a small bowl, mash the avocado with the olive oil and lemon juice. Season with a pinch of salt and pepper.

3. Spread the mashed avocado evenly over the toasted English muffin halves.

4. Top the avocado toast with any desired additional toppings, such as sliced tomatoes, everything bagel seasoning, or red pepper flakes.

This whole grain English muffin with avocado makes a great option for managing type 2 diabetes for a few reasons:

- Whole grain English muffins are a complex carb that is high in fiber, which helps slow the absorption of carbs and stabilize blood sugar levels.

- Avocado is high in healthy monounsaturated fats, which can help improve insulin sensitivity.

- The healthy fats and fiber in avocado also help keep you feeling full and satisfied.

- Lemon juice and optional toppings like tomatoes provide additional nutrients and antioxidants.

This makes a nutritious and filling breakfast or snack. You can adjust the portion size as needed to fit your individual dietary needs for managing type 2 diabetes. Enjoy!

21. Apple Slices with Peanut Butter

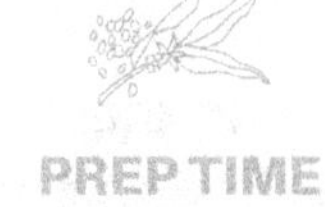

PREP TIME
20 MINUTES

COOK TIME
30 MINUTES

INGREDIENTS :

- 1 medium apple, cored and sliced
- 2 tbsp natural peanut butter (no added sugar)
- Cinnamon (optional)

PROCEDURE :

1. Wash and slice the apple into thin wedges or slices.

2. Spread 1-2 teaspoons of natural peanut butter onto each apple slice.

3. If desired, sprinkle a light dusting of cinnamon over the top of the peanut butter.

That's it! This simple snack is a great option for managing type 2 diabetes for a few reasons:

- Apples are a low-glycemic fruit, meaning they won't spike your blood sugar too much. They are also high in fiber.

- Natural peanut butter is a good source of healthy fats and protein, which can help slow the absorption of carbs from the apple.

- The combination of the apple's fiber and the peanut butter's protein and fat helps keep you feeling full and satisfied.

- Cinnamon may help improve insulin sensitivity.

This makes a nutritious and portable snack. You can adjust the portion sizes to fit your individual dietary needs for managing type 2 diabetes. Enjoy!

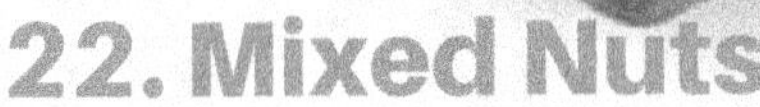

22. Mixed Nuts

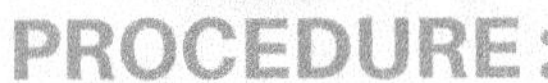

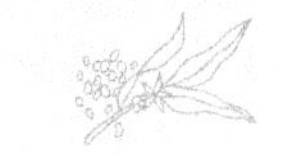

PREP TIME
20 MINUTES

COOK TIME
30 MINUTES

INGREDIENTS:

- 1/4 cup raw, unsalted mixed nuts (such as almonds, walnuts, pecans, cashews)

1. Measure out 1/4 cup of the mixed nuts.

That's it! This simple snack of mixed nuts is an excellent choice for managing type 2 diabetes for several reasons:

- Nuts are high in healthy fats, protein, and fiber, which can help regulate blood sugar levels and keep you feeling full.

- The combination of different nuts provides a variety of beneficial nutrients like magnesium, vitamin E, and antioxidants.

- Nuts have a low glycemic index, meaning they won't cause a rapid spike in blood sugar.

- Unsalted, raw nuts are the healthiest option, as they don't contain added oils, sugars, or salt.

A 1/4 cup serving of mixed nuts is a great portion size to aim for as a snack. You can keep individual servings pre-portioned in small containers or bags for easy, diabetes-friendly snacking on the go.

Remember to pay attention to portion sizes, as nuts are calorie-dense. Adjust the amount as needed to fit your individual dietary requirements for managing type 2 diabetes. Enjoy this simple yet nutritious snack!

23. Celery Sticks with Hummus

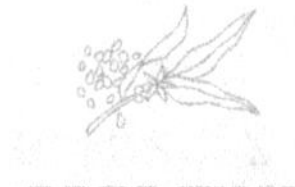

PREP TIME
20 MINUTES

COOK TIME
30 MINUTES

INGREDIENTS :

- 2-3 celery stalks, cut into 4-inch sticks
- 2-3 tablespoons of hummus (look for a brand with minimal added sugars)

PROCEDURE :

1. Wash and cut the celery stalks into 4-inch sticks.

2. Scoop the hummus into a small bowl or ramekin.

3. Dip the celery sticks into the hummus and enjoy.

This celery and hummus snack is an excellent choice for managing type 2 diabetes for several reasons:

- Celery is an extremely low-carb vegetable, providing fiber, vitamins, and minerals without spiking blood sugar.

- Hummus is made from chickpeas, which are a good source of complex carbs, fiber, and protein. The healthy fats from the tahini and olive oil in hummus also help slow the absorption of carbs.

- The combination of the crunchy celery and creamy hummus provides a satisfying texture and flavor.

- Hummus brands that are low in added sugars are a better choice for managing diabetes.

This makes a great snack or appetizer. You can adjust the portion sizes of the celery and hummus to fit your individual dietary needs for managing type 2 diabetes. Enjoy!

24. Hard-Boiled Eggs

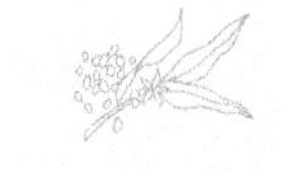

PREP TIME
20 MINUTES

COOK TIME
30 MINUTES

INGREDIENTS:

- 6 large eggs

PROCEDURE:

1. Place the eggs in a single layer in a saucepan and cover with cold water by 1 inch.

2. Bring the water to a boil over high heat.

3. Once the water reaches a full boil, remove the pan from the heat and cover with a lid. Let the eggs sit in the hot water for:
- Soft-boiled: 3-5 minutes
- Hard-boiled: 12 minutes

4. Drain the hot water and cover the eggs with cold water to stop the cooking.

5. Let the eggs sit in the cold water for 5 minutes.

6. Peel the eggs and enjoy as a snack, or store in the refrigerator for up to 1 week.

Hard-boiled eggs are an excellent snack option for managing type 2 diabetes for several reasons:

- Eggs are high in protein, which helps stabilize blood sugar levels and keep you feeling full.
- They contain no carbs, making them a diabetes-friendly food.
- Hard-boiled eggs are portable, easy to prepare, and can be kept on hand for quick snacking.
- Eggs are also a good source of other important nutrients like choline, vitamin D, and antioxidants.

You can enjoy hard-boiled eggs plain, or try adding a sprinkle of salt, pepper, or a small amount of low-fat mayonnaise or mustard for extra flavor. Adjust the portion size as needed to fit your individual dietary requirements for managing type 2 diabetes.

25. Cheese and Whole Grain Crackers

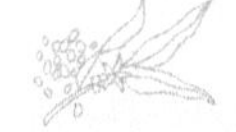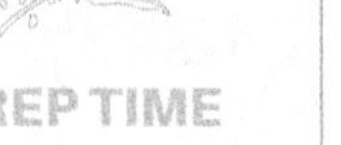

PREP TIME
20 MINUTES

COOK TIME
30 MINUTES

INGREDIENTS :

- 6-8 whole grain crackers (look for ones with at least 3g of fiber per serving)
- 1-2 oz sliced or cubed cheddar, Swiss, or other low-fat cheese
- Optional: grapes, apple slices, or cherry tomatoes

PROCEDURE :

1. Arrange the whole grain crackers on a plate or small board.

2. Top each cracker with a slice or cube of the low-fat cheese.

3. If desired, add a few grapes, apple slices, or cherry tomatoes alongside the crackers and cheese.

This snack of cheese and whole grain crackers is a great option for managing type 2 diabetes for several reasons:

- Whole grain crackers are a complex carb that is high in fiber, which helps slow the absorption of carbs and stabilize blood sugar levels.

- Cheese provides protein and healthy fats to help keep you feeling full and satisfied.

- The optional fruit toppings like grapes or apple slices add natural sweetness and fiber without spiking blood sugar too much.

- The combination of the complex carbs, protein, and healthy fats helps prevent blood sugar spikes and crashes.

This makes a portable and satisfying snack. You can adjust the portion sizes of the crackers and cheese to fit your individual dietary needs for managing type 2 diabetes. Enjoy!

26. Edamame

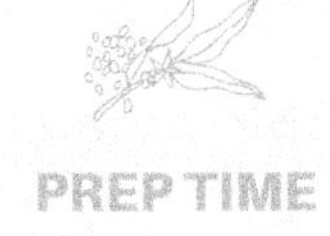

PREP TIME
20 MINUTES

COOK TIME
30 MINUTES

INGREDIENTS:

- 1 cup frozen edamame in the pod

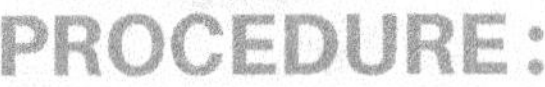

PROCEDURE:

1. Bring a pot of water to a boil.

2. Add the frozen edamame pods and cook for 5-7 minutes until tender.

3. Drain the edamame and sprinkle with a pinch of salt (optional).

4. Serve the edamame warm, in the pod, for snacking.

Edamame is an excellent snack choice for managing type 2 diabetes for several reasons:

- Edamame is a type of immature soybean that is low in carbs and high in fiber and protein. This helps prevent blood sugar spikes.

- The fiber and protein in edamame also help keep you feeling full and satisfied.

- Edamame contains beneficial plant compounds like isoflavones that may help improve insulin sensitivity.

- It's a convenient, portable snack that's easy to prepare.

When enjoying edamame, be mindful of portion sizes. A 1 cup serving of cooked edamame contains around 8 grams of carbs, so adjust the amount based on your individual dietary needs for managing type 2 diabetes.

This simple snack of boiled edamame pods makes a great option to have on hand. You can also experiment with different seasonings like garlic powder, lemon juice, or soy sauce for added flavor. Enjoy!

27. Greek Yogurt with Cucumber Slices

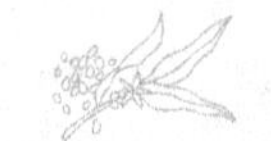

PREP TIME
20 MINUTES

COOK TIME
30 MINUTES

INGREDIENTS:

- 1 cup plain Greek yogurt (full-fat or low-fat)
- 1 medium cucumber, sliced into rounds
- 1 tsp fresh dill (optional)
- Salt and pepper to taste

PROCEDURE:

1. Scoop the Greek yogurt into a small bowl or serving dish.

2. Wash and slice the cucumber into thin rounds.

3. Arrange the cucumber slices around the edge of the yogurt.

4. If desired, sprinkle the fresh dill over the top of the yogurt.

5. Season with a pinch of salt and pepper.

This Greek yogurt and cucumber snack is a great option for managing type 2 diabetes for several reasons:

- Greek yogurt is high in protein, which helps keep you feeling full and satisfied. The protein also helps stabilize blood sugar levels.

- Cucumbers are an extremely low-carb vegetable, providing hydration, fiber, and vitamins without spiking blood sugar.

- The combination of the creamy yogurt and crunchy cucumber provides a refreshing and satisfying texture.

- The optional dill adds flavor without any carbs.

This makes a simple, nutritious, and diabetes-friendly snack. You can adjust the portion sizes of the yogurt and cucumber to fit your individual dietary needs. Enjoy!

28. Kale Chips

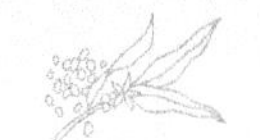

PREP TIME
20 MINUTES

COOK TIME
30 MINUTES

INGREDIENTS:

- 1 bunch of kale, washed and dried thoroughly
- 1-2 tbsp olive oil
- Salt and pepper to taste
- Optional seasonings: garlic powder, onion powder, paprika, cayenne pepper

PROCEDURE:

1. Preheat your oven to 325°F (165°C).

2. Wash the kale and pat it completely dry with paper towels or a clean kitchen towel. Make sure there is no excess moisture on the leaves.

3. Tear or cut the kale leaves into bite-sized pieces, discarding any thick stems.

4. Place the kale pieces in a large bowl and drizzle with the olive oil. Use your hands to massage the oil evenly over the kale.

5. Spread the kale pieces out in a single layer on one or more baking sheets, making sure they are not overlapping.

6. Sprinkle the kale with salt and pepper, and any other desired seasonings.

7. Bake for 12-15 minutes, flipping the kale halfway through, until the chips are crispy and lightly browned.

8. Remove the kale chips from the oven and let them cool completely before serving.

Kale chips make a great snack option for managing type 2 diabetes because:

- Kale is an extremely low-carb, high-fiber vegetable that won't spike blood sugar.
- The healthy fats from the olive oil help slow the absorption of carbs.
- The crunchy texture satisfies the desire for a crispy snack.
- You can customize the seasonings to your taste preferences.

29. Sliced Bell Peppers with Guacamole

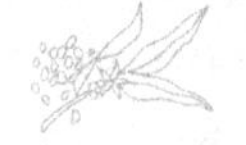 

PREP TIME 20 MINUTES

COOK TIME 30 MINUTES

INGREDIENTS :

- 1 medium bell pepper, sliced into strips
- 2 tablespoons homemade or store-bought guacamole

PROCEDURE :

1. Wash and slice the bell pepper into long, thin strips.
2. Scoop out 2 tablespoons of guacamole and serve alongside the bell pepper strips.

Nutrition Information (per serving):
- Calories: 80
- Total Carbs: 8g
- Fiber: 3g
- Net Carbs: 5g
- Protein: 2g
- Fat: 5g

Why this is a good snack for type 2 diabetes:

- Bell peppers are low in carbs and high in fiber, vitamins, and antioxidants.

- Guacamole is a great source of healthy monounsaturated fats from avocado, which can help manage blood sugar levels.

- The combination of the crunchy bell peppers and creamy guacamole provides a satisfying and balanced snack.

Tips:

- Choose a bell pepper color you enjoy - red, yellow, or orange are all great options.

- Make your own guacamole to control the ingredients and avoid added sugars.

- Pair this snack with a glass of water or unsweetened tea.

30. Almond Butter on Whole Grain Crackers

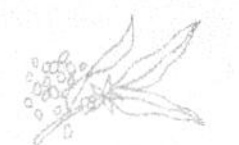

PREP TIME
20 MINUTES

COOK TIME
30 MINUTES

INGREDIENTS:

- 2 tablespoons natural almond butter
- 6-8 whole grain crackers (look for ones high in fiber and low in added sugars)

PROCEDURE:

1. Spread about 1-2 teaspoons of almond butter evenly onto each whole grain cracker.

Nutrition Information (per serving):
- Calories: 150
- Total Carbs: 10g
- Fiber: 3g
- Net Carbs: 7g
- Protein: 5g
- Fat: 11g

Why this is a good snack for type 2 diabetes:

- Almond butter is high in healthy fats and protein, which can help manage blood sugar levels.

- Whole grain crackers provide complex carbs, fiber, and nutrients compared to refined crackers.

- The combination of healthy fats, protein, and complex carbs helps create a balanced snack that won't spike blood sugar too quickly.

Tips:
- Look for crackers with at least 3g of fiber per serving.

- Stick to 1-2 tablespoons of almond butter to keep carbs and calories in check.

- Pair with a glass of water or unsweetened tea for hydration.

31. Veggie Sticks with Low-Fat Dip

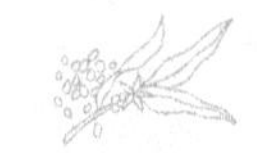

PREP TIME
20 MINUTES

COOK TIME
30 MINUTES

INGREDIENTS :

- 1 cup sliced cucumber
- 1 cup baby carrots
- 1/4 cup low-fat plain Greek yogurt
- 1 tablespoon chopped fresh herbs (such as dill, chives, or parsley)
- 1 teaspoon lemon juice
- Salt and pepper to taste

PROCEDURE :

1. Wash and slice the cucumber into sticks. Rinse and leave the baby carrots whole.

2. In a small bowl, mix together the Greek yogurt, chopped herbs, lemon juice, salt, and pepper.

3. Serve the veggie sticks alongside the low-fat yogurt dip.

Nutrition Information (per serving):
- Calories: 70
- Total Carbs: 8g
- Fiber: 2g
- Net Carbs: 6g
- Protein: 4g
- Fat: 2g

Why this is a good snack for type 2 diabetes:

- Vegetables like cucumbers and carrots are low in carbs and high in fiber, vitamins, and minerals.

- The low-fat Greek yogurt dip provides protein and calcium without added sugars.

- The combination of crunchy veggies and creamy dip makes for a satisfying and balanced snack.

Tips:

- Try other veggie options like celery, bell pepper strips, or cherry tomatoes.

- Experiment with different herb and spice combinations in the dip.

- Pair this snack with a glass of water or unsweetened tea.

32. Trail Mix with Nuts and Seeds

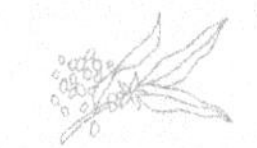 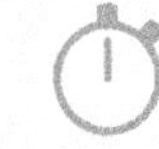

PREP TIME
20 MINUTES

COOK TIME
30 MINUTES

INGREDIENTS:

- 1 cup raw almonds
- 1 cup raw cashews
- 1/2 cup raw pumpkin seeds
- 1/2 cup raw sunflower seeds
- 1/2 cup dried cranberries
- 1/4 cup unsweetened coconut flakes

PROCEDURE:

1. In a large bowl, combine the almonds, cashews, pumpkin seeds, sunflower seeds, dried cranberries, and coconut flakes.

2. Stir the ingredients together until well mixed.

3. Transfer the trail mix to an airtight container or resealable bag.

4. Store at room temperature for up to 2 weeks.

Enjoy this nutritious and satisfying trail mix as a snack on the go or as part of a balanced meal. The combination of nuts, seeds, and dried fruit provides a nice balance of healthy fats, protein, fiber, and carbohydrates.

33. Cherry Tomatoes and Mozzarella

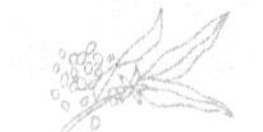 

PREP TIME
20 MINUTES

COOK TIME
30 MINUTES

INGREDIENTS :

- 10-12 cherry tomatoes, halved
- 2 oz fresh mozzarella cheese, cut into bite-sized pieces
- 1 tsp balsamic glaze (optional)
- Fresh basil leaves (optional)
- Salt and pepper to taste

PROCEDURE :

1. Wash the cherry tomatoes and slice them in half.

2. Cut the mozzarella cheese into small cubes or bite-sized pieces.

3. Arrange the tomato halves and mozzarella pieces on a plate or in a small bowl.

4. Drizzle the balsamic glaze over the top, if using.

5. Tear or chop a few fresh basil leaves and sprinkle them over the top (optional).

6. Season with a pinch of salt and pepper.

This cherry tomatoes and mozzarella snack is a great option for managing type 2 diabetes for several reasons:

- Cherry tomatoes are low in carbs and high in fiber, vitamins, and antioxidants.

- Mozzarella cheese provides protein and healthy fats to help stabilize blood sugar levels.

- The combination of the juicy tomatoes, creamy cheese, and optional balsamic glaze and basil creates a flavorful and satisfying snack.

- This snack is easy to prepare and portable, making it a convenient option.

You can adjust the portion sizes of the tomatoes and mozzarella to fit your individual dietary needs for managing type 2 diabetes. Enjoy this simple yet nutritious snack!

34. Whole Grain Rice Cakes with Avocado

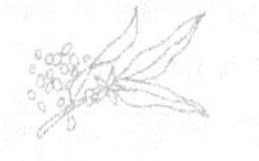 

PREP TIME
20 MINUTES

COOK TIME
30 MINUTES

INGREDIENTS :

- 2 whole grain rice cakes
- 1/2 ripe avocado, mashed
- 1 tbsp olive oil
- Salt and pepper to taste

PROCEDURE :

1. Toast the rice cakes until lightly golden brown.

2. In a small bowl, mash the avocado with a fork until smooth.

3. Drizzle the olive oil over the rice cakes.

4. Spread the mashed avocado evenly over the rice cakes.

5. Season with salt and pepper to taste.

That's it! The creamy avocado pairs perfectly with the crunchy whole grain rice cakes. This makes for a quick, healthy, and satisfying snack or light meal. Enjoy!

35. Sugar Snap Peas and Hummus

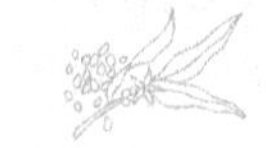

PREP TIME
20 MINUTES

COOK TIME
30 MINUTES

INGREDIENTS:

- 1 cup fresh sugar snap peas, washed and trimmed
- 2-3 tablespoons of hummus (look for a brand with minimal added sugars)

PROCEDURE:

1. Wash and trim the ends off the sugar snap peas.

2. Scoop the hummus into a small bowl or ramekin.

3. Dip the sugar snap peas into the hummus and enjoy.

This sugar snap pea and hummus snack is an excellent choice for managing type 2 diabetes for several reasons:

- Sugar snap peas are a low-carb, high-fiber vegetable that won't spike blood sugar levels.

- Hummus is made from chickpeas, which provide complex carbs, fiber, and protein. The healthy fats from the tahini and olive oil in hummus also help slow the absorption of carbs.

- The combination of the crunchy peas and creamy hummus provides a satisfying texture and flavor.

- Hummus brands that are low in added sugars are a better choice for managing diabetes.

This makes a refreshing and nutritious snack. You can adjust the portion sizes of the peas and hummus to fit your individual dietary needs for managing type 2 diabetes. Enjoy!

36. Blueberries and Almonds

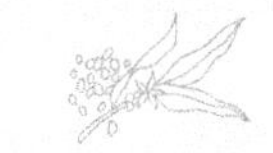

PREP TIME
20 MINUTES

COOK TIME
30 MINUTES

INGREDIENTS :

- 1/2 cup fresh or frozen blueberries
- 2 tbsp raw, unsalted almonds

PROCEDURE :

1. Rinse and gently pat dry the blueberries.

2. Measure out 2 tablespoons of raw, unsalted almonds.

3. Arrange the blueberries and almonds together in a small bowl or container.

This blueberries and almonds snack is an excellent choice for managing type 2 diabetes for several reasons:

- Blueberries are a low-glycemic fruit, meaning they won't cause a rapid spike in blood sugar levels. They are also high in fiber, vitamins, and antioxidants.

- Almonds are a great source of healthy fats, protein, and fiber, which can help regulate blood sugar and keep you feeling full.

- The combination of the sweet blueberries and the crunchy, nutty almonds provides a satisfying and balanced snack.

- Both blueberries and almonds are low in carbs, making them a diabetes-friendly food.

This makes a portable, easy-to-prepare snack that you can enjoy anytime. Be mindful of portion sizes, as nuts are calorie-dense. Adjust the amounts as needed to fit your individual dietary requirements for managing type 2 diabetes. Enjoy!

37. Sliced Pear with Cheese

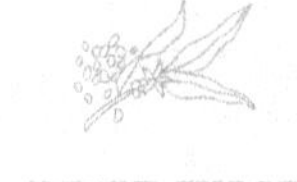

PREP TIME
20 MINUTES

COOK TIME
30 MINUTES

INGREDIENTS :

- 1 ripe but firm pear, cored and sliced
- 2 oz low-fat or reduced-fat cheese (such as cheddar, gouda, or brie)
- Optional: a drizzle of honey or a sprinkle of cinnamon

PROCEDURE :

1. Wash and slice the pear into thin, even slices.

2. Arrange the pear slices on a plate or platter.

3. Cut or crumble the cheese into small pieces and place on top of the pear slices.

4. If desired, drizzle a small amount of honey over the top or sprinkle with a dash of cinnamon.

Nutrition Benefits:

- Pears are a good source of fiber, which can help regulate blood sugar levels. The fiber also promotes feelings of fullness.

- The cheese provides protein, which helps stabilize blood sugar and keeps you feeling satisfied.

- The combination of the fruit and dairy is a balanced snack that contains both carbohydrates and protein.

- This simple snack is low in calories and carbs, making it a diabetes-friendly option.

This easy pear and cheese plate makes for a nutritious, portable, and tasty snack or light meal. It's a great way to incorporate more fruit and dairy into your diet when managing type 2 diabetes.

38. Pumpkin Seeds

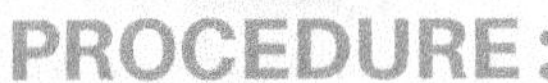

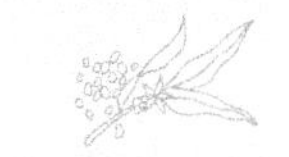

PREP TIME
20 MINUTES

COOK TIME
30 MINUTES

INGREDIENTS:

- 1 cup raw pumpkin seeds, rinsed and dried
- 1 tbsp olive oil or melted butter
- 1 tsp salt (or to taste)
- Optional seasonings: garlic powder, onion powder, chili powder, cumin, paprika, etc.

PROCEDURE:

1. Preheat oven to 325°F (165°C).

2. Spread the rinsed and dried pumpkin seeds in a single layer on a baking sheet.

3. Drizzle the olive oil or melted butter over the seeds and toss to coat evenly.

4. Sprinkle the salt and any other desired seasonings over the seeds and toss to distribute.

5. Roast the seeds for 15-20 minutes, stirring halfway, until lightly golden brown and fragrant.

6. Allow the roasted pumpkin seeds to cool completely before serving. They will continue to crisp up as they cool.

7. Store the roasted pumpkin seeds in an airtight container at room temperature for up to 1 week.

Enjoy the crunchy, nutty, and flavorful roasted pumpkin seeds as a healthy snack or topping for salads, soups, and more. The seasoning options are endless!

39. Radishes with Tzatziki Sauce

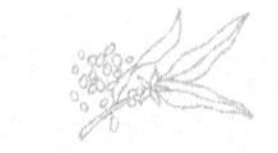 

PREP TIME
20 MINUTES

COOK TIME
30 MINUTES

INGREDIENTS:

- 1 cup sliced radishes
- 1/4 cup plain Greek yogurt
- 1 tbsp finely chopped cucumber
- 1 tsp lemon juice
- 1 tsp chopped fresh dill (or 1/4 tsp dried dill)
- 1 garlic clove, minced
- Salt and pepper to taste

PROCEDURE:

1. Wash and slice the radishes into thin rounds or wedges.

2. In a small bowl, mix together the Greek yogurt, chopped cucumber, lemon juice, dill, and minced garlic. Season with a pinch of salt and pepper.

3. Arrange the sliced radishes on a plate or platter.

4. Serve the tzatziki sauce alongside the radishes for dipping.

This radishes with tzatziki sauce snack is a great option for managing type 2 diabetes for several reasons:

- Radishes are an extremely low-carb, high-fiber vegetable that won't spike blood sugar levels.

- Greek yogurt in the tzatziki sauce provides protein to help stabilize blood sugar.

- The healthy fats from the yogurt and the fiber from the cucumber help slow the absorption of carbs.

- The fresh herbs and lemon juice add flavor without any added sugars.

This makes a refreshing, crunchy, and diabetes-friendly snack. You can adjust the portion sizes of the radishes and tzatziki to fit your individual dietary needs. Enjoy!

40. Roasted Chickpeas

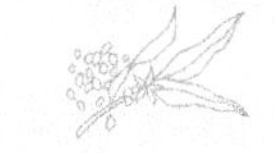 

PREP TIME
20 MINUTES

COOK TIME
30 MINUTES

INGREDIENTS :

- 1 (15 oz) can chickpeas (garbanzo beans), drained and rinsed
- 1 tbsp olive oil
- 1 tsp ground cumin
- 1 tsp paprika
- 1/2 tsp garlic powder
- 1/4 tsp salt

PROCEDURE :

1. Preheat your oven to 400°F (200°C).

2. Pat the drained and rinsed chickpeas dry with a paper towel or clean kitchen towel.

3. In a medium bowl, toss the chickpeas with the olive oil, cumin, paprika, garlic powder, and salt until evenly coated.

4. Spread the seasoned chickpeas in a single layer on a baking sheet lined with parchment paper.

5. Roast the chickpeas for 20-25 minutes, stirring halfway, until they are crispy and golden brown.

6. Allow the roasted chickpeas to cool completely before serving.

Nutrition Benefits:

- Chickpeas are a great source of fiber, protein, and complex carbohydrates, which can help manage blood sugar levels.

- The spices and seasonings add flavor without adding extra carbs or sugar.

- Roasting the chickpeas makes them crispy and crunchy, providing a satisfying snack.

- Chickpeas are low in calories and high in nutrients, making them a diabetes-friendly option.

These roasted chickpeas make for a delicious, crunchy, and nutritious snack that can help manage type 2 diabetes. They are portable, easy to prepare, and can be enjoyed on their own or as a topping for salads, soups, or other dishes.

41. Grilled Chicken Caesar Salad

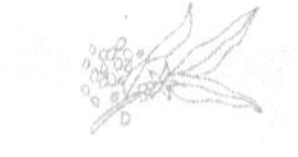

PREP TIME
20 MINUTES

COOK TIME
30 MINUTES

INGREDIENTS:

- 4 oz boneless, skinless chicken breast
- 1 tbsp olive oil
- 1 tsp lemon juice
- Salt and pepper to taste
- 4 cups romaine lettuce, chopped
- 2 tbsp grated Parmesan cheese
- 2 tbsp low-fat or light Caesar dressing

PROCEDURE:

1. Preheat grill or grill pan to medium-high heat.

2. Brush the chicken breast with olive oil and season with salt and pepper.

3. Grill the chicken for 4-5 minutes per side, or until cooked through. Let the chicken rest for 5 minutes, then slice or chop it.

4. In a large salad bowl, combine the chopped romaine lettuce, grilled chicken, Parmesan cheese, and Caesar dressing. Toss gently to coat.

Nutrition Benefits:

- Grilled chicken is a lean protein that won't spike blood sugar levels.

- Romaine lettuce is low in carbs and high in fiber, vitamins, and minerals.

- Parmesan cheese provides protein and calcium without a lot of carbs or fat.

- The Caesar dressing is a lower-carb option compared to many other salad dressings.

This grilled chicken Caesar salad is a balanced, diabetes-friendly meal that provides a good source of protein, fiber, and healthy fats. The combination of greens, lean protein, and a light dressing makes it a satisfying and blood sugar-friendly option.

To further enhance the diabetes-friendly aspects, you can use a homemade low-carb Caesar dressing or opt for a store-bought light or reduced-fat version. You can also add extra vegetables like cherry tomatoes or cucumber slices to boost the nutrient content.

42. Spinach Salad with Walnuts and Goat Cheese

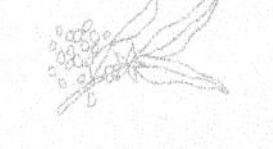 

INGREDIENTS:

- 5 oz baby spinach leaves, washed and dried
- 2 tbsp crumbled goat cheese
- 2 tbsp chopped walnuts
- 1 tbsp olive oil
- 1 tbsp balsamic vinegar
- 1 tsp Dijon mustard
- 1 tsp honey
- Salt and pepper to taste

PROCEDURE:

1. In a large salad bowl, combine the spinach leaves, crumbled goat cheese, and chopped walnuts.

2. In a small bowl, whisk together the olive oil, balsamic vinegar, Dijon mustard, and honey until well combined. Season with salt and pepper.

3. Drizzle the dressing over the spinach salad and toss gently to coat.

Nutrition Benefits:

- Spinach is packed with vitamins, minerals, and antioxidants, and is low in carbs, making it an excellent choice for managing diabetes.

- Walnuts provide healthy fats, fiber, and protein to help stabilize blood sugar levels.

- Goat cheese is a good source of protein and calcium, and has a lower fat and calorie content compared to many other cheeses.

- The olive oil and balsamic vinegar dressing is a simple, diabetes-friendly way to add healthy fats and flavor to the salad.

This spinach salad with walnuts and goat cheese is a nutritious, balanced, and flavorful option that can be enjoyed as a main dish or side salad when managing type 2 diabetes. The combination of greens, healthy fats, and protein makes it a satisfying and blood sugar-friendly meal.

43. Greek Salad with Feta and Olives

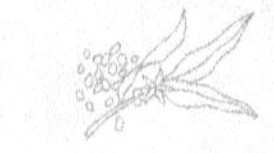

PREP TIME
20 MINUTES

COOK TIME
30 MINUTES

INGREDIENTS :

- 5 oz mixed greens (such as romaine, spinach, and arugula)
- 1/2 cup diced cucumber
- 1/2 cup cherry tomatoes, halved
- 1/4 cup crumbled feta cheese
- 2 tbsp kalamata olives, pitted and halved
- 1 tbsp olive oil
- 1 tbsp red wine vinegar
- 1 tsp dried oregano
- Salt and pepper to taste

PROCEDURE :

1. In a large salad bowl, combine the mixed greens, diced cucumber, cherry tomatoes, crumbled feta cheese, and kalamata olives.

2. In a small bowl, whisk together the olive oil, red wine vinegar, and dried oregano. Season with a pinch of salt and pepper.

3. Drizzle the dressing over the salad and toss gently to coat the ingredients.

Nutrition Benefits:

- Mixed greens are low in carbs and high in fiber, vitamins, and minerals.

- Cucumber and tomatoes provide additional nutrients and fiber without a lot of carbs.

- Feta cheese is a good source of protein and calcium without a lot of carbs.

- Kalamata olives add healthy fats and a flavorful punch.

- The olive oil and red wine vinegar dressing is a diabetes-friendly way to add flavor without added sugars.

This Greek salad with feta and olives is a balanced, nutrient-rich meal or snack that can help manage type 2 diabetes. The combination of greens, vegetables, cheese, and a light dressing makes it a satisfying and blood sugar-friendly option.

To further enhance the diabetes-friendly aspects, you can use a homemade low-carb dressing or opt for a store-bought light or reduced-sugar version. You can also add additional vegetables like bell peppers or onions to boost the nutrient content.

44. Quinoa and Black Bean Salad

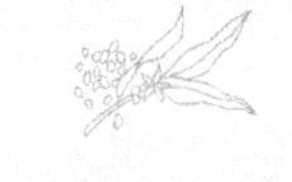

PREP TIME
20 MINUTES

COOK TIME
30 MINUTES

INGREDIENTS:

- 1 cup cooked quinoa, cooled
- 1 (15 oz) can black beans, rinsed and drained
- 1 cup diced cucumber
- 1 cup diced tomatoes
- 1/2 cup diced red onion
- 2 tbsp chopped fresh cilantro
- 2 tbsp lime juice
- 1 tbsp olive oil
- 1 tsp ground cumin
- 1/4 tsp salt
- 1/4 tsp black pepper

PROCEDURE:

1. In a large bowl, combine the cooked and cooled quinoa, black beans, diced cucumber, diced tomatoes, diced red onion, and chopped cilantro.

2. In a small bowl, whisk together the lime juice, olive oil, cumin, salt, and black pepper.

3. Pour the dressing over the quinoa and bean mixture and toss gently to coat.

4. Refrigerate the salad for at least 30 minutes to allow the flavors to meld. Serve chilled or at room temperature.

Nutrition Benefits:

- Quinoa is a whole grain that is high in protein, fiber, and complex carbohydrates.

- Black beans are a great source of plant-based protein and fiber.

- Vegetables like cucumber, tomatoes, and onion add vitamins, minerals, and antioxidants.

- The lime juice, olive oil, and spices provide flavor without added sugars.

This quinoa and black bean salad is a nutritious, balanced, and flavorful dish that can be enjoyed as a main course, side dish, or even a snack. It's a great option for those looking to incorporate more plant-based, high-fiber foods into their diet.

You can customize the salad by adding other vegetables, herbs, or even a small amount of crumbled feta or avocado. This salad is also very versatile - it can be served chilled, at room temperature, or even slightly warmed.

45. Kale and Apple Salad with Lemon Vinaigrette

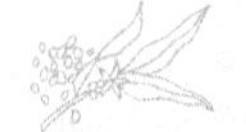 

PREP TIME
20 MINUTES

COOK TIME
30 MINUTES

INGREDIENTS :

- 4 cups chopped kale, stems removed
- 1 medium apple, cored and thinly sliced
- 2 tbsp chopped walnuts
- 1 tbsp crumbled feta cheese
- 2 tbsp fresh lemon juice
- 1 tbsp olive oil
- 1 tsp Dijon mustard
- 1 tsp honey
- Salt and pepper to taste

PROCEDURE :

1. In a large salad bowl, combine the chopped kale, sliced apple, walnuts, and feta cheese.

2. In a small bowl, whisk together the lemon juice, olive oil, Dijon mustard, and honey until well combined. Season with a pinch of salt and pepper.

3. Drizzle the lemon vinaigrette over the kale and apple salad and toss gently to coat the ingredients.

Nutrition Benefits:

- Kale is a nutrient-dense leafy green that is low in carbs and high in fiber, vitamins, and antioxidants.

- Apples are a low-glycemic fruit that provide fiber and natural sweetness.

- Walnuts add healthy fats, protein, and fiber to help stabilize blood sugar levels.

- Feta cheese provides protein and calcium without a lot of carbs.

- The lemon vinaigrette is a low-carb, diabetes-friendly dressing that adds flavor without added sugars.

This kale and apple salad with lemon vinaigrette is a balanced, nutrient-rich meal or snack that can help manage type 2 diabetes. The combination of greens, fruit, nuts, and a light dressing makes it a satisfying and blood sugar-friendly option.

To further enhance the diabetes-friendly aspects, you can use a homemade low-carb vinaigrette or opt for a store-bought light or reduced-sugar version. You can also add additional vegetables like bell peppers or cherry tomatoes to boost the nutrient content.

46. Cobb Salad with Turkey and Avocado

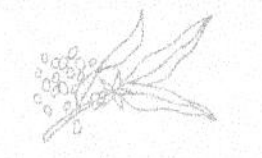 

PREP TIME
20 MINUTES

COOK TIME
30 MINUTES

INGREDIENTS:

- 5 oz mixed greens (such as romaine, spinach, and arugula)
- 3 oz cooked turkey breast, diced
- 1/2 avocado, diced
- 2 hard-boiled eggs, chopped
- 2 tbsp crumbled blue cheese
- 2 tbsp chopped tomatoes
- 2 tbsp chopped cucumber
- 2 tbsp low-fat or light ranch dressing

PROCEDURE:

1. In a large salad bowl, arrange the mixed greens as the base.

2. Top the greens with the diced turkey, avocado, chopped hard-boiled eggs, crumbled blue cheese, chopped tomatoes, and chopped cucumber.

3. Drizzle the low-fat or light ranch dressing over the salad and toss gently to combine.

Nutrition Benefits:

- Mixed greens are low in carbs and high in fiber, vitamins, and minerals.

- Turkey is a lean protein that won't spike blood sugar levels.

- Avocado provides healthy fats and fiber to help stabilize blood sugar.Hard-boiled eggs add protein without carbs.

- Blue cheese provides flavor and a small amount of protein without a lot of carbs.The low-fat or light ranch dressing is a diabetes-friendly option.

This Cobb salad with turkey and avocado is a balanced, nutrient-dense meal that can help manage type 2 diabetes. The combination of greens, lean protein, healthy fats, and a light dressing makes it a satisfying and blood sugar-friendly option.

To further enhance the diabetes-friendly aspects, you can use a homemade low-carb ranch dressing or opt for a store-bought light or reduced-fat version. You can also add additional vegetables like bell peppers or cucumber to boost the nutrient content.

47. Broccoli Salad with Sunflower Seeds

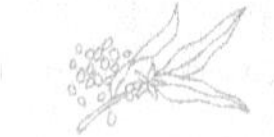

PREP TIME	COOK TIME
20 MINUTES	30 MINUTES

INGREDIENTS :

- 4 cups broccoli florets, chopped
- 1/2 cup diced red onion
- 1/2 cup shredded cheddar cheese
- 1/4 cup roasted sunflower seeds
- 3 tbsp low-fat or light mayonnaise
- 2 tbsp apple cider vinegar
- 1 tbsp honey
- Salt and pepper to taste

PROCEDURE :

1. In a large bowl, combine the chopped broccoli florets, diced red onion, shredded cheddar cheese, and roasted sunflower seeds.

2. In a small bowl, whisk together the mayonnaise, apple cider vinegar, and honey until well combined. Season with a pinch of salt and pepper.

3. Pour the dressing over the broccoli salad and toss gently to coat the ingredients.

4. Refrigerate the salad for at least 30 minutes to allow the flavors to meld.. Serve chilled or at room temperature.

Nutrition Benefits:

- Broccoli is a nutrient-dense vegetable that is low in carbs and high in fiber, vitamins, and antioxidants.

- Red onion adds crunch and flavor without a lot of carbs.Cheddar cheese provides protein and calcium.

- Sunflower seeds are a good source of healthy fats, protein, and fiber.

- The mayonnaise, vinegar, and honey dressing adds flavor without a lot of added sugars.

This broccoli salad with sunflower seeds is a nutritious, balanced, and flavorful dish that can be enjoyed as a side dish or a light main course. It's a great option for those looking to incorporate more vegetables and healthy fats into their diet.

48. Tuna Salad with Mixed Greens

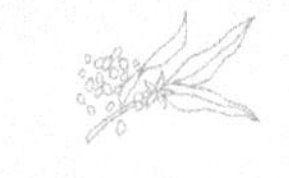

PREP TIME
20 MINUTES

COOK TIME
30 MINUTES

INGREDIENTS :

- 5 oz mixed greens (such as spinach, arugula, and romaine)
- 3 oz canned tuna, drained
- 2 tbsp diced celery
- 2 tbsp diced red onion
- 1 tbsp chopped parsley
- 1 tbsp olive oil
- 1 tbsp lemon juice
- 1 tsp Dijon mustard
- Salt and pepper to taste

PROCEDURE :

1. In a medium bowl, combine the drained tuna, diced celery, diced red onion, and chopped parsley.

2. In a small bowl, whisk together the olive oil, lemon juice, and Dijon mustard. Season with a pinch of salt and pepper.

3. Arrange the mixed greens on a plate or in a salad bowl.

4. Top the greens with the tuna salad mixture and drizzle the dressing over the top.

5. Toss the salad gently to coat the greens with the tuna and dressing.

Nutrition Benefits:

- Mixed greens are low in carbs and high in fiber, vitamins, and minerals.
- Tuna is a lean protein that is low in carbs and high in healthy omega-3 fatty acids.
- Celery and onion add crunch and flavor without a lot of carbs.
- The olive oil and lemon juice dressing is a diabetes-friendly way to add healthy fats and flavor.

This tuna salad with mixed greens is a balanced, nutrient-dense meal that can help manage type 2 diabetes. The combination of lean protein, greens, and a light dressing makes it a satisfying and blood sugar-friendly option.

To further enhance the diabetes-friendly aspects, you can use a homemade low-carb dressing or opt for a store-bought light or reduced-sugar version. You can also add additional vegetables like cherry tomatoes or cucumber to boost the nutrient content.

49. Roasted Beet and Arugula Salad

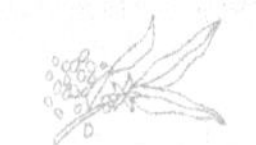

PREP TIME
20 MINUTES

COOK TIME
30 MINUTES

INGREDIENTS:

- 3 medium beets, peeled and cut into 1-inch cubes
- 1 tbsp olive oil
- Salt and pepper to taste
- 5 oz baby arugula
- 2 tbsp crumbled feta cheese
- 2 tbsp chopped walnuts
- 2 tbsp balsamic vinegar
- 1 tsp Dijon mustard
- 1 tsp honey

PROCEDURE:

1. Preheat your oven to 400°F (200°C).

2. Toss the cubed beets with the olive oil and season with salt and pepper.

3. Spread the seasoned beets on a baking sheet and roast for 20-25 minutes, or until tender and lightly caramelized.

4. Allow the roasted beets to cool slightly.

5. In a large salad bowl, combine the baby arugula, roasted beets, crumbled feta cheese, and chopped walnuts.

6. In a small bowl, whisk together the balsamic vinegar, Dijon mustard, and honey.

7. Drizzle the balsamic vinaigrette over the salad and toss gently to coat.

Nutrition Benefits:

- Beets are a low-glycemic root vegetable that are high in fiber, vitamins, and antioxidants.
- Arugula is a nutrient-dense leafy green that is low in carbs and high in fiber.
- Feta cheese provides protein and calcium without a lot of carbs.
- Walnuts add healthy fats, protein, and fiber to help stabilize blood sugar levels.
- The balsamic vinaigrette is a diabetes-friendly dressing that adds flavor without added sugars.

This roasted beet and arugula salad is a balanced, nutrient-rich meal or snack that can help manage type 2 diabetes. The combination of roasted vegetables, greens, cheese, and nuts makes it a satisfying and blood sugar-friendly option.

50. Chickpea and Tomato Salad

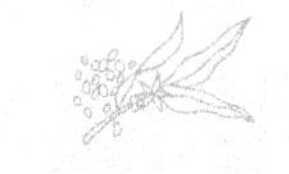

PREP TIME
20 MINUTES

COOK TIME
30 MINUTES

INGREDIENTS:

- 1 (15 oz) can chickpeas (garbanzo beans), drained and rinsed
- 1 cup cherry tomatoes, halved
- 1/2 cup diced cucumber
- 1/4 cup diced red onion
- 2 tbsp chopped fresh parsley
- 2 tbsp olive oil
- 1 tbsp red wine vinegar
- 1 tsp Dijon mustard
- 1 tsp honey
- Salt and pepper to taste

PROCEDURE:

1. In a large bowl, combine the drained and rinsed chickpeas, halved cherry tomatoes, diced cucumber, diced red onion, and chopped parsley.

2. In a small bowl, whisk together the olive oil, red wine vinegar, Dijon mustard, and honey. Season with a pinch of salt and pepper.

3. Pour the dressing over the chickpea and tomato mixture and toss gently to coat.

4. Refrigerate the salad for at least 30 minutes to allow the flavors to meld. Serve chilled or at room temperature.

Nutrition Benefits:

- Chickpeas are a good source of plant-based protein, fiber, and complex carbohydrates.
- Cherry tomatoes and cucumber provide vitamins, minerals, and antioxidants.
- Red onion adds flavor and crunch without a lot of carbs.
- The olive oil, vinegar, and mustard dressing is a diabetes-friendly way to add flavor without added sugars.

This chickpea and tomato salad is a nutritious, balanced, and flavorful dish that can be enjoyed as a main course, side dish, or even a snack. It's a great option for those looking to incorporate more plant-based, high-fiber foods into their diet.

You can customize the salad by adding other vegetables, such as bell peppers or avocado, or by using a different type of vinegar or herbs in the dressing. This salad is also very versatile - it can be served chilled, at room temperature, or even slightly warmed.

51. Spinach and Strawberry Salad

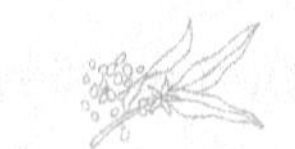

PREP TIME
20 MINUTES

COOK TIME
30 MINUTES

INGREDIENTS :

- 5 oz baby spinach leaves, washed and dried
- 1 cup fresh strawberries, sliced
- 2 tbsp crumbled feta cheese
- 2 tbsp chopped walnuts
- 1 tbsp balsamic vinegar
- 1 tsp olive oil
- 1 tsp Dijon mustard
- 1 tsp honey
- Salt and pepper to taste

PROCEDURE :

1. In a large salad bowl, combine the baby spinach leaves, sliced strawberries, crumbled feta cheese, and chopped walnuts.

2. In a small bowl, whisk together the balsamic vinegar, olive oil, Dijon mustard, and honey until well combined. Season with a pinch of salt and pepper.

3. Drizzle the dressing over the salad and toss gently to coat the ingredients.

Nutrition Benefits:

- Spinach is low in carbs and high in fiber, vitamins, and minerals, making it an excellent choice for managing diabetes.
- Strawberries are a low-glycemic fruit that are high in fiber and antioxidants.
- Feta cheese provides protein and calcium without a lot of carbs.
- Walnuts add healthy fats, protein, and fiber to help stabilize blood sugar levels.
- The balsamic vinegar and Dijon mustard-based dressing is low in carbs and calories.

This spinach and strawberry salad is a balanced, diabetes-friendly meal or snack that is packed with nutrients and fiber to help manage blood sugar levels. The combination of greens, fruit, cheese, and nuts makes it a satisfying and flavorful option.

To further enhance the diabetes-friendly aspects, you can use a homemade low-carb dressing or opt for a store-bought light or reduced-sugar version. You can also add additional vegetables like cucumber or bell peppers to boost the nutrient content.

52. Caprese Salad

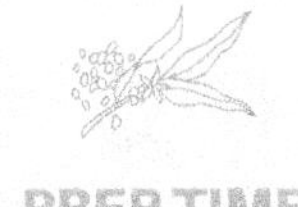 

PREP TIME
20 MINUTES

COOK TIME
30 MINUTES

INGREDIENTS :

- 8 oz fresh mozzarella cheese, sliced
- 1 cup cherry tomatoes, halved
- 1/4 cup fresh basil leaves, torn
- 1 tbsp balsamic glaze (or reduced-balsamic vinegar)
- 1 tbsp olive oil
- 1/4 tsp salt
- 1/4 tsp black pepper

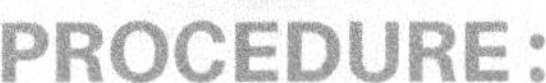

PROCEDURE :

1. Arrange the sliced mozzarella cheese and halved cherry tomatoes on a serving platter or plate.

2. Sprinkle the torn fresh basil leaves over the top.

3. Drizzle the balsamic glaze and olive oil over the salad.

4. Season with salt and black pepper.

Nutrition Benefits:

- Fresh mozzarella cheese is a good source of protein and calcium without a lot of carbs.
- Cherry tomatoes are a low-glycemic fruit that are high in vitamins, minerals, and antioxidants.
- Fresh basil adds flavor without any carbs.
- The balsamic glaze and olive oil dressing provides healthy fats and a touch of sweetness without added sugars.

This Caprese salad is a simple, yet flavorful and diabetes-friendly option. The combination of creamy mozzarella, juicy tomatoes, and fragrant basil makes it a refreshing and satisfying meal or snack.

To further enhance the diabetes-friendly aspects, you can use a homemade balsamic glaze or reduced-balsamic vinegar. You can also add other low-carb vegetables like sliced cucumber or bell peppers to the salad.

This Caprese salad is a great way to incorporate healthy fats, protein, and fresh produce into your diet while managing type 2 diabetes. The minimal ingredients and easy preparation make it a convenient and versatile option.

53. Cucumber and Dill Salad

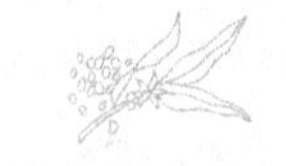

PREP TIME
20 MINUTES

COOK TIME
30 MINUTES

INGREDIENTS :

- 5 oz mixed greens (such as romaine, spinach, and arugula)
- 3 oz cooked turkey breast, diced
- 1/2 avocado, diced
- 2 hard-boiled eggs, chopped
- 2 tbsp crumbled blue cheese
- 2 tbsp chopped tomatoes
- 2 tbsp chopped cucumber
- 2 tbsp low-fat or light ranch dressing

PROCEDURE :

1. In a medium bowl, combine the sliced cucumber, thinly sliced red onion, and chopped fresh dill.

2. In a small bowl, whisk together the white wine vinegar, olive oil, lemon juice, salt, and black pepper.

3. Pour the dressing over the cucumber and onion mixture and toss gently to coat.

4. Refrigerate the salad for at least 30 minutes to allow the flavors to meld. Serve chilled or at room temperature.

Nutrition Benefits:

- Cucumbers are a low-calorie, low-carb vegetable that are high in water content and provide hydration.
- Red onion adds flavor and crunch without a lot of carbs.
- Fresh dill is a flavorful herb that doesn't contain any carbs.
- The vinegar, oil, and lemon juice dressing is a diabetes-friendly way to add flavor without added sugars.

This cucumber and dill salad is a refreshing, low-carb, and nutrient-dense option that can help manage type 2 diabetes. The combination of crisp vegetables, fresh herbs, and a light dressing makes it a satisfying and blood sugar-friendly side dish or snack.

To further enhance the diabetes-friendly aspects, you can use a homemade low-carb dressing or opt for a store-bought light or reduced-sugar version. You can also add other low-carb vegetables like cherry tomatoes or bell peppers to boost the nutrient content.

54. Roasted Vegetable Salad

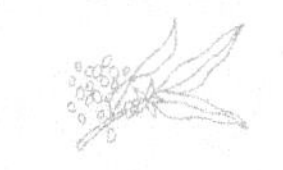

PREP TIME
20 MINUTES

COOK TIME
30 MINUTES

INGREDIENTS :

- 1 cup cubed butternut squash
- 1 cup broccoli florets
- 1 cup sliced zucchini
- 1 tbsp olive oil
- Salt and pepper to taste
- 5 oz mixed greens (such as spinach, arugula, and kale)
- 2 tbsp crumbled feta cheese
- 2 tbsp toasted pumpkin seeds
- 2 tbsp balsamic vinaigrette (or use a homemade low-carb version)

PROCEDURE :

1. Preheat your oven to 400°F (200°C).

2. Toss the cubed butternut squash, broccoli florets, and sliced zucchini with the olive oil. Season with a pinch of salt and pepper.

3. Spread the seasoned vegetables on a baking sheet and roast for 20-25 minutes, or until tender and lightly caramelized.

4. Allow the roasted vegetables to cool slightly.

5. In a large salad bowl, combine the mixed greens, roasted vegetables, crumbled feta cheese, and toasted pumpkin seeds.

6. Drizzle the balsamic vinaigrette over the salad and toss gently to coat the ingredients.

Nutrition Benefits:

- Butternut squash, broccoli, and zucchini are low-glycemic vegetables that are high in fiber, vitamins, and antioxidants.
- Mixed greens are a nutrient-dense base that is low in carbs and high in fiber.
- Feta cheese provides protein and calcium without a lot of carbs.
- Pumpkin seeds add healthy fats, protein, and fiber to help stabilize blood sugar levels.
- The balsamic vinaigrette is a diabetes-friendly dressing that adds flavor without added sugars.

This roasted vegetable salad is a balanced, nutrient-rich meal or snack that can help manage type 2 diabetes. The combination of roasted vegetables, greens, cheese, and a light dressing makes it a satisfying and blood sugar-friendly option.

55. Salmon and Avocado Salad

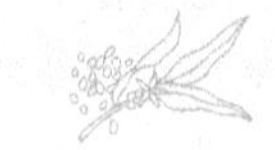

PREP TIME
20 MINUTES

COOK TIME
30 MINUTES

INGREDIENTS :

- 4 oz cooked salmon, flaked
- 1/2 avocado, diced
- 2 cups mixed greens (such as spinach, arugula, and kale)
- 1/4 cup diced cucumber
- 2 tbsp chopped red onion
- 1 tbsp olive oil
- 1 tbsp lemon juice
- 1 tsp Dijon mustard
- Salt and pepper to taste

PROCEDURE :

1. In a large salad bowl, combine the flaked cooked salmon, diced avocado, mixed greens, diced cucumber, and chopped red onion.

2. In a small bowl, whisk together the olive oil, lemon juice, and Dijon mustard. Season with a pinch of salt and pepper.

3. Drizzle the dressing over the salmon and avocado salad and toss gently to coat the ingredients.

Nutrition Benefits:

- Salmon is a lean protein that is high in heart-healthy omega-3 fatty acids.
- Avocado provides healthy monounsaturated fats and fiber to help stabilize blood sugar levels.
- Mixed greens are low in carbs and high in fiber, vitamins, and minerals.
- Cucumber and red onion add crunch and flavor without a lot of carbs.
- The olive oil and lemon juice dressing is a diabetes-friendly way to add flavor without added sugars.

This salmon and avocado salad is a balanced, nutrient-dense meal that can help manage type 2 diabetes. The combination of lean protein, healthy fats, and a light dressing makes it a satisfying and blood sugar-friendly option.

To further enhance the diabetes-friendly aspects, you can use a homemade low-carb dressing or opt for a store-bought light or reduced-sugar version. You can also add additional vegetables like cherry tomatoes or bell peppers to boost the nutrient content.

56. Lentil and Feta Salad

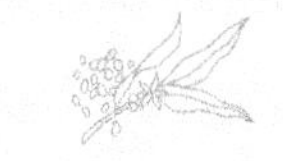

INGREDIENTS :

- 1 cup cooked lentils, cooled
- 1/2 cup diced cucumber
- 1/4 cup crumbled feta cheese
- 2 tbsp chopped fresh parsley
- 1 tbsp olive oil
- 1 tbsp red wine vinegar
- 1 tsp Dijon mustard
- 1 tsp lemon juice
- Salt and pepper to taste

PROCEDURE :

1. In a large bowl, combine the cooked and cooled lentils, diced cucumber, crumbled feta cheese, and chopped parsley.

2. In a small bowl, whisk together the olive oil, red wine vinegar, Dijon mustard, and lemon juice. Season with a pinch of salt and pepper.

3. Pour the dressing over the lentil and feta salad and toss gently to coat the ingredients.

4. Refrigerate the salad for at least 30 minutes to allow the flavors to meld. Serve chilled or at room temperature.

Nutrition Benefits:

- Lentils are a great source of plant-based protein, fiber, and complex carbohydrates.
- Cucumber adds crunch and hydration without a lot of carbs.
- Feta cheese provides protein and calcium without a lot of carbs.
- The olive oil, vinegar, and lemon juice dressing is a diabetes-friendly way to add flavor without added sugars.

This lentil and feta salad is a balanced, nutrient-dense meal or snack that can help manage type 2 diabetes. The combination of protein-rich lentils, healthy fats, and a light dressing makes it a satisfying and blood sugar-friendly option.

To further enhance the diabetes-friendly aspects, you can use a homemade low-carb dressing or opt for a store-bought light or reduced-sugar version. You can also add additional vegetables like cherry tomatoes or bell peppers to boost the nutrient content.

57. Asian Chicken Salad

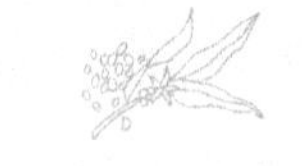

PREP TIME
20 MINUTES

COOK TIME
30 MINUTES

INGREDIENTS :

- 4 oz cooked chicken breast, shredded or diced
- 2 cups shredded cabbage (or coleslaw mix)
- 1/2 cup shredded carrots
- 1/4 cup sliced green onions
- 2 tbsp chopped cilantro
- 2 tbsp rice vinegar
- 1 tbsp sesame oil
- 1 tsp low-sodium soy sauce
- 1 tsp Dijon mustard
- 1 tsp honey
- Salt and pepper to taste

PROCEDURE :

1. In a large salad bowl, combine the shredded chicken, shredded cabbage, shredded carrots, sliced green onions, and chopped cilantro.

2. In a small bowl, whisk together the rice vinegar, sesame oil, soy sauce, Dijon mustard, and honey. Season with a pinch of salt and pepper.

3. Pour the dressing over the salad and toss gently to coat the ingredients.

Nutrition Benefits:

- Chicken is a lean protein that won't spike blood sugar levels.
- Cabbage and carrots are low-carb vegetables that are high in fiber and vitamins.
- Green onions and cilantro add flavor without carbs.
- The rice vinegar, sesame oil, and Dijon mustard dressing is a diabetes-friendly way to add Asian-inspired flavors without added sugars.

This Asian chicken salad is a balanced, flavorful, and diabetes-friendly meal or snack. The combination of lean protein, crunchy vegetables, and a light dressing makes it a satisfying and blood sugar-friendly option.

To further enhance the diabetes-friendly aspects, you can use a homemade low-carb dressing or opt for a store-bought light or reduced-sugar version. You can also add other low-carb vegetables like bell peppers or snow peas to boost the nutrient content.

58. Watermelon and Feta Salad

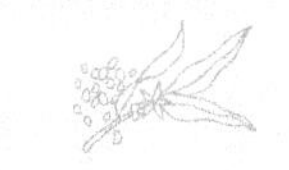

PREP TIME
20 MINUTES

COOK TIME
30 MINUTES

INGREDIENTS:

- 2 cups cubed watermelon
- 1/2 cup crumbled feta cheese
- 1/4 cup thinly sliced red onion
- 2 tbsp chopped fresh mint
- 1 tbsp balsamic glaze
- 1 tbsp olive oil
- 1 tbsp lime juice
- Salt and pepper to taste

PROCEDURE:

1. In a large bowl, combine the cubed watermelon, crumbled feta cheese, thinly sliced red onion, and chopped fresh mint.

2. In a small bowl, whisk together the balsamic glaze, olive oil, and lime juice. Season with a pinch of salt and pepper.

3. Drizzle the dressing over the watermelon and feta salad and toss gently to coat the ingredients.

4. Refrigerate the salad for at least 15 minutes to allow the flavors to meld.

Nutrition Benefits:
- Watermelon is a low-glycemic fruit that is high in water content and provides hydration.
- Feta cheese is a good source of protein and calcium without a lot of carbs.
- Red onion adds flavor and crunch without a lot of carbs.
- Fresh mint provides a refreshing flavor without any carbs.
- The balsamic glaze and olive oil dressing is a diabetes-friendly way to add flavor without added sugars.

This watermelon and feta salad is a refreshing, low-carb, and nutrient-dense option that can help manage type 2 diabetes. The combination of sweet fruit, salty cheese, and a light dressing makes it a satisfying and blood sugar-friendly side dish or snack.

To further enhance the diabetes-friendly aspects, you can use a homemade low-carb balsamic glaze or opt for a store-bought reduced-sugar version. You can also add other low-carb vegetables like cucumber or cherry tomatoes to boost the nutrient content.

59. Cauliflower Rice Salad

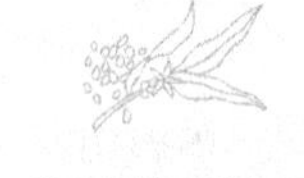

PREP TIME
20 MINUTES

COOK TIME
30 MINUTES

INGREDIENTS:

- 3 cups riced cauliflower (about 1 small head of cauliflower, riced)
- 1/2 cup diced cucumber
- 1/2 cup diced tomatoes
- 1/4 cup diced red onion
- 2 tbsp chopped fresh parsley
- 2 tbsp olive oil
- 2 tbsp lemon juice
- 1 tsp Dijon mustard
- 1/4 tsp salt
- 1/4 tsp black pepper

PROCEDURE:

1. In a large bowl, combine the riced cauliflower, diced cucumber, diced tomatoes, diced red onion, and chopped parsley.

2. In a small bowl, whisk together the olive oil, lemon juice, Dijon mustard, salt, and black pepper.

3. Pour the dressing over the cauliflower rice salad and toss gently to coat the ingredients.

4. Refrigerate the salad for at least 30 minutes to allow the flavors to meld. Serve chilled or at room temperature.

Nutrition Benefits:

- Cauliflower rice is a low-carb, high-fiber alternative to traditional rice.
- Cucumber, tomatoes, and red onion add crunch, flavor, and additional nutrients without a lot of carbs.
- Fresh parsley provides antioxidants and flavor without any carbs.
- The olive oil, lemon juice, and Dijon mustard dressing is a diabetes-friendly way to add healthy fats and flavor.

This cauliflower rice salad is a nutritious, balanced, and flavorful dish that can be enjoyed as a side dish or a light main course. It's a great option for those looking to incorporate more low-carb, vegetable-based foods into their diet.

You can customize the salad by adding other vegetables, such as bell peppers or avocado, or by using a different type of herb or citrus juice in the dressing. This salad is also very versatile - it can be served chilled, at room temperature, or even slightly warmed.

60. Arugula and Walnut Salad

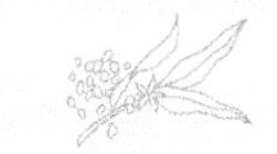

PREP TIME
20 MINUTES

COOK TIME
30 MINUTES

INGREDIENTS:

- 5 oz baby arugula
- 1/4 cup chopped walnuts
- 2 tbsp crumbled feta cheese
- 1 tbsp olive oil
- 1 tbsp balsamic vinegar
- 1 tsp Dijon mustard
- 1 tsp honey
- Salt and pepper to taste

PROCEDURE:

1. In a large salad bowl, combine the baby arugula, chopped walnuts, and crumbled feta cheese.

2. In a small bowl, whisk together the olive oil, balsamic vinegar, Dijon mustard, and honey. Season with a pinch of salt and pepper.

3. Drizzle the dressing over the arugula salad and toss gently to coat the ingredients.

Nutrition Benefits:

- Arugula is a nutrient-dense leafy green that is low in carbs and high in fiber, vitamins, and antioxidants.

- Walnuts provide healthy fats, protein, and fiber to help stabilize blood sugar levels.

- Feta cheese adds protein and calcium without a lot of carbs.

- The olive oil, balsamic vinegar, and Dijon mustard dressing is a diabetes-friendly way to add flavor without added sugars.

This arugula and walnut salad is a balanced, nutrient-rich meal or snack that can help manage type 2 diabetes. The combination of greens, healthy fats, and a light dressing makes it a satisfying and blood sugar-friendly option.

To further enhance the diabetes-friendly aspects, you can use a homemade low-carb dressing or opt for a store-bought light or reduced-sugar version. You can also add additional vegetables like cherry tomatoes or cucumber to boost the nutrient content.

61. Chicken Vegetable Soup

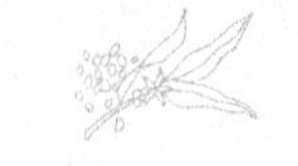

PREP TIME
20 MINUTES

COOK TIME
30 MINUTES

INGREDIENTS :

- 1 lb boneless, skinless chicken breasts, cut into 1-inch pieces
- 1 tbsp olive oil
- 1 onion, diced
- 3 carrots, peeled and sliced
- 2 celery stalks, sliced
- 3 garlic cloves, minced
- 6 cups low-sodium chicken broth
- 1 bay leaf
- 1 tsp dried thyme
- Salt and pepper to taste
- 2 cups chopped kale or spinach
- 1 cup frozen peas

PROCEDURE :

1. In a large pot or Dutch oven, heat the olive oil over medium heat. Add the chicken and cook for 2-3 minutes until lightly browned.

2. Add the onion, carrots, celery and garlic. Cook for 5 minutes, stirring occasionally, until the vegetables start to soften.

3. Pour in the chicken broth and add the bay leaf and thyme. Season with salt and pepper.

4. Bring the soup to a boil, then reduce heat and let simmer for 15-20 minutes.

5. Stir in the kale/spinach and frozen peas. Cook for 5 more minutes until the greens are wilted and the peas are heated through.

6. Remove the bay leaf before serving. Taste and adjust seasoning as needed.

Serve the chicken vegetable soup hot. Enjoy!

62. Lentil Soup

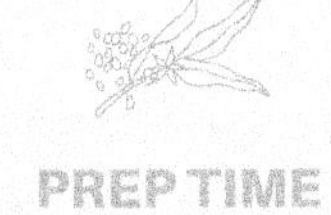

PREP TIME
20 MINUTES

COOK TIME
30 MINUTES

INGREDIENTS :

- 1 cup dry brown or green lentils, rinsed
- 4 cups low-sodium chicken or vegetable broth
- 1 cup diced tomatoes (canned or fresh)
- 1 cup diced carrots
- 1/2 cup diced onion
- 2 cloves garlic, minced
- 1 tsp ground cumin
- 1 tsp dried oregano
- 1/4 tsp cayenne pepper (optional)
- Salt and pepper to taste

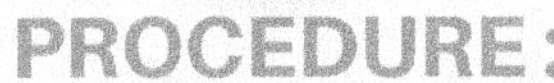

PROCEDURE :

1. In a large pot, combine the rinsed lentils and broth. Bring to a boil over high heat.

2. Once boiling, reduce the heat to medium-low and let the lentils simmer for 15-20 minutes, or until tender.

3. Add the diced tomatoes, carrots, onion, and garlic to the pot. Stir in the cumin, oregano, and cayenne pepper (if using).

4. Continue simmering the soup for an additional 10-15 minutes, or until the vegetables are tender.

5. Season the lentil soup with salt and pepper to taste. Serve the lentil soup hot.

Nutrition Benefits:

- Lentils are a great source of plant-based protein, fiber, and complex carbohydrates, which can help manage blood sugar levels.
- Carrots and tomatoes provide additional vitamins, minerals, and antioxidants without a lot of carbs.
- The low-sodium broth and lack of heavy cream or other high-fat ingredients keep the soup diabetes-friendly.
- The spices add flavor without adding any carbs.

This lentil soup is a nutritious, filling, and diabetes-friendly option. The combination of protein-rich lentils, vegetables, and a flavorful broth makes it a satisfying and blood sugar-friendly meal.

To further enhance the diabetes-friendly aspects, you can use a low-sodium or no-salt-added broth and adjust the amount of spices to your preference. You can also add additional vegetables, such as spinach or zucchini, to boost the nutrient content.

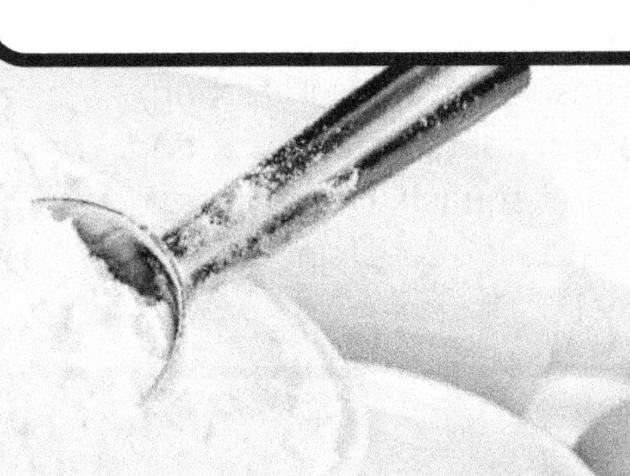

63. Butternut Squash Soup

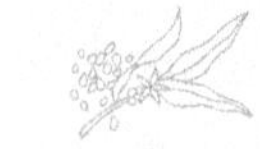

PREP TIME
20 MINUTES

COOK TIME
30 MINUTES

INGREDIENTS :

- 1 medium butternut squash, peeled, seeded, and cubed (about 4 cups)
- 1 cup low-sodium chicken or vegetable broth
- 1 cup unsweetened almond milk
- 1 tbsp olive oil
- 1 onion, diced
- 2 cloves garlic, minced
- 1 tsp ground cinnamon
- 1/4 tsp ground nutmeg
- Salt and pepper to taste

PROCEDURE :

1. In a large pot or Dutch oven, heat the olive oil over medium heat. Add the diced onion and sauté for 3-4 minutes, until translucent.

2. Add the minced garlic and sauté for an additional minute.

3. Add the cubed butternut squash, chicken or vegetable broth, and unsweetened almond milk to the pot. Bring the mixture to a boil.

4. Reduce the heat to medium-low and let the soup simmer for 20-25 minutes, or until the squash is very soft.

5. Using an immersion blender or regular blender, puree the soup until smooth.

6. Stir in the ground cinnamon and nutmeg. Season with salt and pepper to taste. Serve the butternut squash soup hot.

Nutrition Benefits:
- Butternut squash is a low-glycemic, nutrient-dense vegetable that is high in fiber, vitamins, and antioxidants.
- Unsweetened almond milk is a diabetes-friendly alternative to regular milk, as it is low in carbs and high in healthy fats.
- The small amount of olive oil and lack of heavy cream or other high-fat ingredients keep the soup low in calories and carbs.
- The warm spices, such as cinnamon and nutmeg, add flavor without any carbs.

This butternut squash soup is a comforting, nutrient-dense, and diabetes-friendly option. The combination of sweet squash, creamy broth, and warming spices makes it a satisfying and blood sugar-friendly meal

64. Minestrone Soup

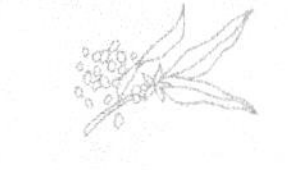

PREP TIME
20 MINUTES

COOK TIME
30 MINUTES

INGREDIENTS :

- 1 tbsp olive oil
- 1 onion, diced
- 3 garlic cloves, minced
- 2 carrots, peeled and diced
- 2 celery stalks, diced
- 1 zucchini, diced
- 1 (15 oz) can diced tomatoes
- 4 cups low-sodium chicken or vegetable broth
- 1 (15 oz) can kidney beans, rinsed and drained
- 1 cup frozen green beans
- 1 cup small whole wheat pasta (such as ditalini or elbow)
- 2 cups chopped kale or spinach
- 1 tsp dried oregano
- 1 tsp dried basil
- Salt and pepper to taste

PROCEDURE :

1. In a large pot, heat the olive oil over medium heat. Add the onion and garlic and cook for 2-3 minutes until fragrant.

2. Add the carrots, celery, and zucchini. Cook for 5 minutes, stirring occasionally, until the vegetables start to soften.

3. Pour in the diced tomatoes and broth. Bring the soup to a boil.

4. Reduce heat and let the soup simmer for 10 minutes.

5. Stir in the kidney beans, green beans, pasta, kale/spinach, oregano, and basil. Season with salt and pepper.

6. Continue simmering for 10-15 more minutes, until the pasta is tender and the vegetables are cooked through.

7. Taste and adjust seasonings as needed.

Serve the minestrone soup hot. This soup is packed with fiber, protein, and nutrients that are great for managing type 2 diabetes.

65. Tomato Basil Soup

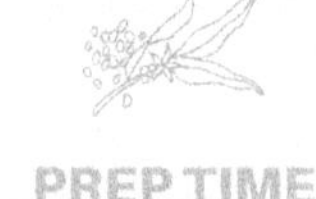

PREP TIME
20 MINUTES

COOK TIME
30 MINUTES

INGREDIENTS:

- 1 (28 oz) can diced tomatoes
- 1 cup low-sodium chicken or vegetable broth
- 1/2 cup unsweetened almond milk
- 2 tbsp fresh basil, chopped
- 1 tsp garlic powder
- 1/4 tsp onion powder
- Salt and pepper to taste

PROCEDURE:

1. In a medium saucepan, combine the diced tomatoes, chicken or vegetable broth, and unsweetened almond milk.

2. Bring the mixture to a simmer over medium heat, stirring occasionally.

3. Once simmering, reduce the heat to low and stir in the chopped fresh basil, garlic powder, and onion powder.

4. Let the soup simmer for 10-15 minutes, allowing the flavors to meld.

5. Using an immersion blender or regular blender, puree the soup until smooth.

6. Season the soup with salt and pepper to taste.

7. Serve the tomato basil soup hot.

Nutrition Benefits:

- Tomatoes are a low-glycemic fruit that are high in vitamins, minerals, and antioxidants.
- Unsweetened almond milk is a diabetes-friendly alternative to regular milk, as it is low in carbs and high in healthy fats.
- Fresh basil adds flavor without any carbs.
- The small amount of broth and lack of heavy cream or other high-fat dairy keeps the soup low in calories and carbs.

This tomato basil soup is a flavorful, nutrient-dense, and diabetes-friendly option. The combination of juicy tomatoes, fragrant basil, and a creamy broth makes it a satisfying and blood sugar-friendly meal or snack.

66. Beef and Barley Soup

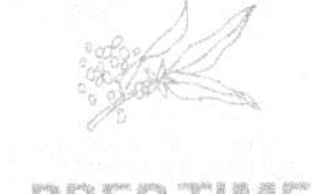

PREP TIME
20 MINUTES

COOK TIME
30 MINUTES

INGREDIENTS :

- 1 lb lean beef stew meat, cut into 1-inch cubes
- 2 tbsp olive oil
- 1 onion, diced
- 3 carrots, peeled and sliced
- 2 celery stalks, sliced
- 3 garlic cloves, minced
- 6 cups low-sodium beef or chicken broth
- 1 cup pearl barley
- 1 (14.5 oz) can diced tomatoes
- 2 tsp dried thyme
- 1 bay leaf
- Salt and pepper to taste
- 2 cups chopped kale or spinach (optional)

PROCEDURE :

1. In a large pot or Dutch oven, heat the olive oil over medium-high heat. Add the beef cubes and brown on all sides, about 5 minutes total. Remove beef to a plate.

2. Reduce heat to medium and add the onion, carrots, celery, and garlic to the pot. Cook for 5-7 minutes, stirring occasionally, until the vegetables start to soften.

3. Pour in the broth and add the barley, diced tomatoes, thyme, and bay leaf. Season with salt and pepper.

4. Bring the soup to a boil, then reduce heat and let it simmer for 45-60 minutes, until the barley is tender.

5. Add the browned beef back to the pot and continue simmering for 15-20 more minutes.

6. Stir in the chopped kale or spinach (if using) and cook for 5 more minutes until the greens are wilted.

7. Remove the bay leaf. Taste and adjust seasoning as needed.

Serve the beef and barley soup hot. This hearty soup is high in fiber, protein, and complex carbs, making it a great option for managing type 2 diabetes. The barley provides soluble fiber to help regulate blood sugar levels.

67. Cauliflower Soup

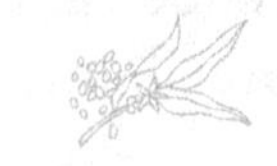

PREP TIME
20 MINUTES

COOK TIME
30 MINUTES

INGREDIENTS:

- 1 tbsp olive oil
- 1 onion, diced
- 3 garlic cloves, minced
- 1 head of cauliflower, cut into florets (about 6 cups)
- 4 cups low-sodium chicken or vegetable broth
- 1 cup unsweetened almond milk
- 1 tsp dried thyme
- 1/2 tsp ground cumin
- Salt and pepper to taste
- 2 tbsp grated Parmesan cheese (optional)
- Chopped parsley for garnish (optional)

PROCEDURE:

1. In a large pot or Dutch oven, heat the olive oil over medium heat. Add the onion and garlic and cook for 2-3 minutes until fragrant.

2. Add the cauliflower florets and broth. Bring the mixture to a boil, then reduce heat and let it simmer for 15-20 minutes, until the cauliflower is very soft.

3. Remove the pot from heat and use an immersion blender to puree the soup until smooth. Alternatively, you can transfer the soup in batches to a regular blender and blend until smooth.

4. Stir in the almond milk, thyme, and cumin. Season with salt and pepper to taste.

5. Return the soup to low heat and let it gently simmer for 5 more minutes to allow the flavors to meld.

6. Ladle the cauliflower soup into bowls. Top with a sprinkle of Parmesan cheese and chopped parsley, if desired.

This creamy cauliflower soup is low in carbs and high in fiber, making it an excellent choice for managing type 2 diabetes. The almond milk provides creaminess without added sugar.

68. Split Pea Soup

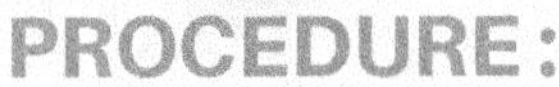

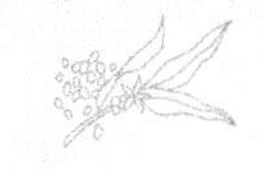

PREP TIME
20 MINUTES

COOK TIME
30 MINUTES

INGREDIENTS :

- 1 tbsp olive oil
- 1 onion, diced
- 3 carrots, peeled and diced
- 2 celery stalks, diced
- 3 garlic cloves, minced
- 1 lb dried split peas, rinsed
- 6 cups low-sodium chicken or vegetable broth
- 1 bay leaf
- 1 tsp dried thyme
- Salt and pepper to taste
- 2 cups chopped kale or spinach (optional)

PROCEDURE :

1. In a large pot or Dutch oven, heat the olive oil over medium heat. Add the onion, carrots, celery, and garlic. Cook for 5-7 minutes, stirring occasionally, until the vegetables start to soften.

2. Add the rinsed split peas, broth, bay leaf, and thyme. Season with salt and pepper.

3. Bring the soup to a boil, then reduce heat and let it simmer for 45-60 minutes, stirring occasionally, until the split peas are very soft and the soup has thickened.

4. Remove the bay leaf. Use an immersion blender or regular blender to puree about half of the soup, leaving some texture.

5. Stir in the chopped kale or spinach (if using) and cook for 5 more minutes until the greens are wilted.

6. Taste and adjust seasoning as needed.

Serve the split pea soup hot. This soup is high in fiber, protein, and complex carbs, making it a great option for managing type 2 diabetes. The fiber and protein help to slow the absorption of carbs and keep blood sugar levels stable.

69. Zucchini and Spinach Soup

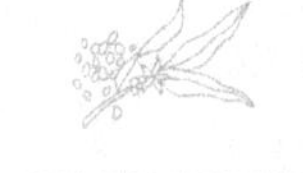

PREP TIME
20 MINUTES

COOK TIME
30 MINUTES

INGREDIENTS :

- 1 tbsp olive oil
- 1 onion, diced
- 3 garlic cloves, minced
- 3 medium zucchini, diced
- 4 cups low-sodium chicken or vegetable broth
- 2 cups fresh spinach, chopped
- 1 tsp dried basil
- 1/2 tsp dried oregano
- Salt and pepper to taste
- 2 tbsp grated Parmesan cheese (optional)

PROCEDURE :

1. In a large pot or Dutch oven, heat the olive oil over medium heat. Add the onion and garlic and cook for 2-3 minutes until fragrant.

2. Add the diced zucchini and chicken/vegetable broth. Bring the mixture to a boil.

3. Reduce heat and let the soup simmer for 15-20 minutes, until the zucchini is very soft.

4. Remove the pot from heat and use an immersion blender to puree the soup until smooth. Alternatively, you can transfer the soup in batches to a regular blender and blend until smooth.

5. Stir in the chopped spinach, basil, and oregano. Season with salt and pepper to taste.

6. Return the soup to low heat and let it simmer for 5 more minutes, until the spinach is wilted.

7. Ladle the zucchini and spinach soup into bowls. Top with a sprinkle of Parmesan cheese, if desired.

This creamy, veggie-packed soup is low in carbs and high in fiber, making it an excellent choice for managing type 2 diabetes. The zucchini and spinach provide vitamins, minerals, and antioxidants.

70. Turkey Chili

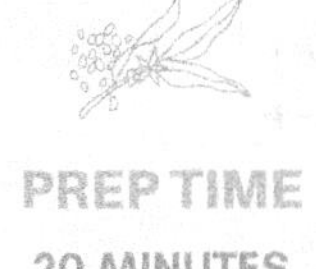 

PREP TIME
20 MINUTES

COOK TIME
30 MINUTES

INGREDIENTS :

- 1 lb ground turkey
- 1 tbsp olive oil
- 1 onion, diced
- 3 garlic cloves, minced
- 2 bell peppers, diced
- 2 cans (15 oz each) no-salt-added diced tomatoes
- 1 can (15 oz) no-salt-added kidney beans, rinsed and drained
- 1 can (15 oz) no-salt-added black beans, rinsed and drained
- 2 tbsp chili powder
- 1 tsp ground cumin
- 1 tsp dried oregano
- 1/2 tsp cayenne pepper (optional, for spice)
- Salt and pepper to taste
- Chopped cilantro for garnish (optional)

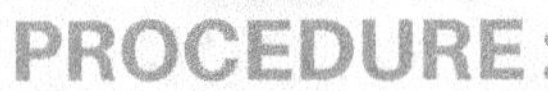

PROCEDURE :

1. In a large pot or Dutch oven, cook the ground turkey over medium-high heat, breaking it up with a wooden spoon, until browned, about 5-7 minutes. Drain any excess fat.

2. Reduce heat to medium and add the olive oil, onion, garlic, and bell peppers. Cook for 5-7 minutes, stirring occasionally, until the vegetables start to soften.

3. Stir in the diced tomatoes, kidney beans, black beans, chili powder, cumin, oregano, and cayenne (if using). Season with salt and pepper.

4. Bring the chili to a boil, then reduce heat and let it simmer for 20-25 minutes, stirring occasionally, until thickened.

5. Taste and adjust seasonings as needed.

6. Serve the turkey chili hot, garnished with chopped cilantro if desired.

This turkey chili is high in protein, fiber, and complex carbs, making it a great option for managing type 2 diabetes. The beans and vegetables provide nutrients while keeping the carb content in check.

71. Broccoli Cheddar Soup

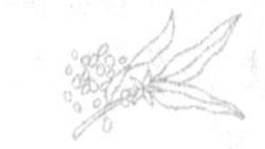

PREP TIME
20 MINUTES

COOK TIME
30 MINUTES

INGREDIENTS :

- 2 cups chopped broccoli florets
- 1 cup low-sodium chicken or vegetable broth
- 1 cup unsweetened almond milk
- 1/2 cup shredded low-fat cheddar cheese
- 2 tbsp butter
- 2 tbsp all-purpose flour
- 1 tsp Dijon mustard
- 1/4 tsp garlic powder
- 1/4 tsp onion powder
- Salt and pepper to taste

PROCEDURE :

1. In a medium saucepan, bring the broth and almond milk to a simmer over medium heat.

2. Add the chopped broccoli florets and cook for 5-7 minutes, or until the broccoli is tender.

3. In a separate small saucepan, melt the butter over medium heat. Whisk in the flour and cook for 1-2 minutes to create a roux.

4. Gradually whisk the roux into the simmering broth and almond milk mixture. Cook, stirring frequently, until the soup thickens slightly, about 5 minutes.

5. Remove the soup from heat and stir in the shredded cheddar cheese, Dijon mustard, garlic powder, and onion powder. Season with salt and pepper to taste.

6. Serve the broccoli cheddar soup hot.

Nutrition Benefits:

- Broccoli is a low-carb, high-fiber vegetable that is packed with vitamins and minerals.
- Low-fat cheddar cheese provides protein and calcium without a lot of carbs.
- Almond milk is a diabetes-friendly alternative to regular milk, as it is low in carbs and high in healthy fats.
- The small amount of flour used to thicken the soup is balanced by the other low-carb ingredients.

This broccoli cheddar soup is a comforting and diabetes-friendly option that can be enjoyed as a main dish or a side. The combination of nutrient-dense broccoli, melted cheese, and a creamy broth makes it a satisfying and blood sugar-friendly meal.

72. Mushroom Barley Soup

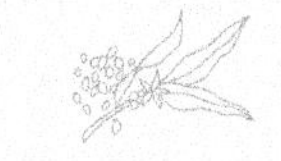 

PREP TIME
20 MINUTES

COOK TIME
30 MINUTES

INGREDIENTS:

- 2 tbsp olive oil
- 1 onion, diced
- 3 garlic cloves, minced
- 8 oz cremini or button mushrooms, sliced
- 1 cup pearl barley, rinsed
- 6 cups low-sodium beef or vegetable broth
- 1 (14.5 oz) can diced tomatoes
- 2 carrots, peeled and sliced
- 2 celery stalks, sliced
- 1 tsp dried thyme
- 1 bay leaf
- Salt and pepper to taste
- Chopped parsley for garnish (optional)

PROCEDURE:

1. In a large pot or Dutch oven, heat the olive oil over medium heat. Add the onion and cook for 3-4 minutes until translucent.

2. Stir in the garlic and mushrooms. Cook for 5-7 minutes, until the mushrooms are softened.

3. Add the pearl barley, broth, diced tomatoes, carrots, celery, thyme, and bay leaf. Season with salt and pepper.

4. Bring the soup to a boil, then reduce heat and let it simmer for 45-60 minutes, until the barley is tender.

5. Remove the bay leaf. Taste and adjust seasoning as needed.

6. Ladle the mushroom barley soup into bowls and garnish with chopped parsley if desired.

This hearty, earthy soup is packed with fiber, protein, and nutrients. The barley provides complex carbs to help keep blood sugar levels stable. You can use a variety of mushrooms like shiitake, oyster, or portobello for extra flavor.

This soup makes a great main dish or side. It's also easy to customize by adding other vegetables like spinach, kale, or zucchini.

73. Vegetable Beef Soup

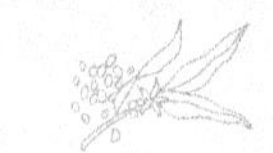

PREP TIME
20 MINUTES

COOK TIME
30 MINUTES

INGREDIENTS :

- 1 lb lean beef stew meat, cut into 1-inch cubes
- 2 tbsp olive oil
- 1 onion, diced
- 3 garlic cloves, minced
- 4 cups low-sodium beef broth
- 1 (14.5 oz) can diced tomatoes
- 2 carrots, peeled and sliced
- 2 celery stalks, sliced
- 1 cup frozen green beans
- 1 cup frozen peas
- 1 tsp dried thyme
- 1 bay leaf
- Salt and pepper to taste
- Chopped parsley for garnish (optional)

PROCEDURE :

1. In a large pot or Dutch oven, heat the olive oil over medium-high heat. Add the beef cubes and brown on all sides, about 5 minutes total. Remove the beef to a plate.

2. Reduce heat to medium and add the onion and garlic to the pot. Cook for 3-4 minutes until fragrant.

3. Pour in the beef broth and add the diced tomatoes, carrots, celery, green beans, peas, thyme, and bay leaf. Season with salt and pepper.

4. Bring the soup to a boil, then reduce heat and let it simmer for 45-60 minutes, until the beef is very tender.

5. Remove the bay leaf. Taste and adjust seasoning as needed.

6. Ladle the vegetable beef soup into bowls and garnish with chopped parsley if desired.

This hearty, veggie-packed soup is a great way to enjoy lean protein, complex carbs, and a variety of nutrients. The long simmer time allows the flavors to meld together perfectly.

You can customize the soup by using different vegetables or adding potatoes, barley, or pasta. This makes a satisfying and comforting meal.

74. Cabbage Soup

PREP TIME
20 MINUTES

COOK TIME
30 MINUTES

INGREDIENTS :

- 1 tbsp olive oil
- 1 onion, diced
- 3 garlic cloves, minced
- 1 head of green cabbage, cored and chopped
- 4 cups low-sodium chicken or vegetable broth
- 1 (15 oz) can diced tomatoes
- 2 carrots, peeled and sliced
- 2 celery stalks, sliced
- 1 tsp dried thyme
- 1 bay leaf
- Salt and pepper to taste
- Chopped parsley for garnish (optional)

PROCEDURE :

1. In a large pot or Dutch oven, heat the olive oil over medium heat. Add the onion and garlic and cook for 2-3 minutes until fragrant.

2. Add the chopped cabbage, broth, diced tomatoes, carrots, celery, thyme, and bay leaf. Season with salt and pepper.

3. Bring the soup to a boil, then reduce heat and let it simmer for 30-40 minutes, until the vegetables are very tender.

4. Remove the bay leaf. Taste and adjust seasoning as needed.

5. Ladle the cabbage soup into bowls and garnish with chopped parsley if desired.

This simple cabbage soup is packed with fiber, vitamins, and antioxidants from the cabbage, carrots, and tomatoes. It's a great low-calorie, low-carb option that can be enjoyed on its own or as a side dish.

You can customize the soup by adding other vegetables like potatoes, zucchini, or spinach. You can also stir in some cooked chicken or beans for extra protein.

75. Lemon Chicken Orzo Soup

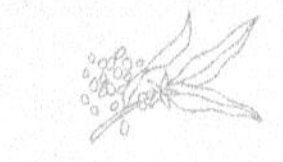 

PREP TIME
20 MINUTES

COOK TIME
30 MINUTES

INGREDIENTS :

- 1 lb boneless, skinless chicken breasts, cut into 1-inch pieces
- 2 tbsp olive oil
- 1 onion, diced
- 3 garlic cloves, minced
- 8 cups low-sodium chicken broth
- 1 cup uncooked orzo pasta
- 2 cups chopped kale or spinach
- Juice of 1 lemon
- 2 tsp lemon zest
- 1 tsp dried thyme
- Salt and pepper to taste
- Chopped fresh parsley for garnish

PROCEDURE :

1. In a large pot or Dutch oven, heat the olive oil over medium-high heat. Add the chicken and cook for 3-4 minutes, until lightly browned.

2. Add the onion and garlic to the pot and cook for 2-3 minutes, until fragrant.

3. Pour in the chicken broth and bring the mixture to a boil. Stir in the orzo pasta and reduce heat to medium-low. Simmer for 10-12 minutes, until the orzo is tender.

4. Stir in the chopped kale/spinach, lemon juice, lemon zest, and thyme. Season with salt and pepper to taste.

5. Continue simmering for 5 more minutes, until the greens are wilted.

6. Ladle the lemon chicken orzo soup into bowls and garnish with chopped fresh parsley.

This bright and flavorful soup is a great way to enjoy lean protein, whole grains, and nutrient-dense greens. The lemon adds a refreshing zing that complements the chicken and orzo.

76. Spicy Black Bean Soup

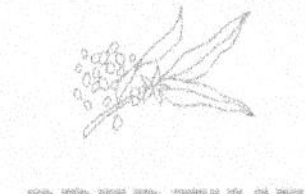

PREP TIME
20 MINUTES

COOK TIME
30 MINUTES

INGREDIENTS :

- 2 tbsp olive oil
- 1 onion, diced
- 3 garlic cloves, minced
- 2 tsp ground cumin
- 1 tsp chili powder
- 1/2 tsp smoked paprika
- 1/4 tsp cayenne pepper (optional, for extra spice)
- 2 (15 oz) cans no-salt-added black beans, rinsed and drained
- 4 cups low-sodium chicken or vegetable broth
- 1 (14.5 oz) can no-salt-added diced tomatoes
- 1 bay leaf
- Salt and pepper to taste
- Chopped cilantro for garnish (optional)
- Lime wedges for serving

PROCEDURE :

1. In a large pot or Dutch oven, heat the olive oil over medium heat. Add the onion and cook for 3-4 minutes until translucent.

2. Stir in the garlic, cumin, chili powder, smoked paprika, and cayenne (if using). Cook for 1 minute until fragrant.

3. Add the black beans, broth, diced tomatoes, and bay leaf. Season with salt and pepper.

4. Bring the soup to a boil, then reduce heat and let it simmer for 20-25 minutes, stirring occasionally, until slightly thickened.

5. Remove the bay leaf. Use an immersion blender to puree about half of the soup, leaving some texture. Alternatively, you can transfer 2-3 cups of the soup to a regular blender and blend until smooth, then return it to the pot.

6. Taste and adjust seasoning as needed.

7. Ladle the spicy black bean soup into bowls and garnish with chopped cilantro, if desired. Serve with lime wedges.

This hearty, protein-packed soup is an excellent choice for managing type 2 diabetes. The black beans provide fiber and complex carbs, while the spices add flavor without added sugar.

77. Carrot Ginger Soup

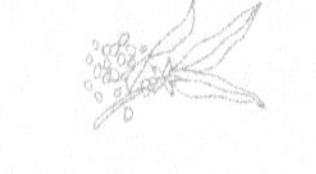

PREP TIME
20 MINUTES

COOK TIME
30 MINUTES

INGREDIENTS:

- 1 tbsp olive oil
- 1 onion, diced
- 3 garlic cloves, minced
- 1 tbsp grated fresh ginger
- 1 lb carrots, peeled and sliced
- 4 cups low-sodium chicken or vegetable broth
- 1 cup unsweetened almond milk
- 1 tsp ground cumin
- 1/4 tsp cayenne pepper (optional)
- Salt and pepper to taste
- Chopped fresh parsley for garnish (optional)

PROCEDURE:

1. In a large pot or Dutch oven, heat the olive oil over medium heat. Add the onion and cook for 3-4 minutes until translucent.

2. Stir in the garlic and grated ginger. Cook for 1 minute until fragrant.

3. Add the sliced carrots and chicken/vegetable broth. Bring the mixture to a boil.

4. Reduce heat and let the soup simmer for 20-25 minutes, until the carrots are very soft.

5. Remove the pot from heat and use an immersion blender to puree the soup until smooth. Alternatively, you can transfer the soup in batches to a regular blender and blend until creamy.

6. Stir in the unsweetened almond milk, cumin, and cayenne (if using). Season with salt and pepper to taste.

7. Return the soup to low heat and let it simmer for 5 more minutes to allow the flavors to meld.

8. Ladle the carrot ginger soup into bowls and garnish with chopped fresh parsley if desired.

This creamy, nutrient-dense soup is an excellent choice for managing type 2 diabetes. The carrots provide fiber and beta-carotene, while the ginger adds anti-inflammatory benefits. The almond milk keeps the carb count low.

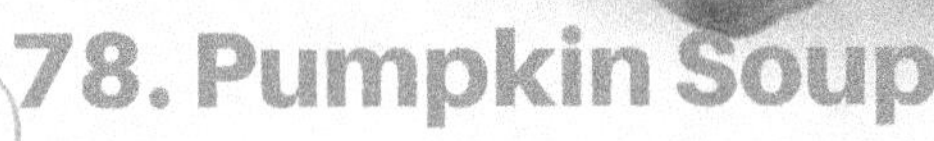

78. Pumpkin Soup

PREP TIME
20 MINUTES

COOK TIME
30 MINUTES

INGREDIENTS:

- 2 tbsp olive oil
- 1 onion, diced
- 3 garlic cloves, minced
- 1 (15 oz) can pure pumpkin puree
- 4 cups low-sodium chicken or vegetable broth
- 1 cup unsweetened almond milk
- 1 tsp ground cinnamon
- 1/2 tsp ground ginger
- 1/4 tsp ground nutmeg
- 1/4 tsp cayenne pepper (optional)
- Salt and pepper to taste
- Chopped fresh parsley or chives for garnish (optional)
- Toasted pumpkin seeds (optional)

PROCEDURE:

1. In a large pot or Dutch oven, heat the olive oil over medium heat. Add the onion and cook for 3-4 minutes until translucent.

2. Stir in the garlic and cook for 1 minute until fragrant.

3. Add the pumpkin puree, broth, almond milk, cinnamon, ginger, nutmeg, and cayenne (if using). Season with salt and pepper.

4. Bring the soup to a simmer, then reduce heat and let it cook for 15-20 minutes, stirring occasionally, until heated through.

5. Use an immersion blender to puree the soup until smooth. Alternatively, you can transfer the soup in batches to a regular blender and blend until creamy.

6. Taste and adjust seasoning as needed.

7. Ladle the pumpkin soup into bowls and garnish with chopped parsley or chives, and toasted pumpkin seeds if desired.

This creamy, spiced pumpkin soup is perfect for fall. The pumpkin provides fiber, vitamins, and antioxidants, while the almond milk keeps it dairy-free and low in carbs. Enjoy this comforting soup as a main dish or appetizer.

79. White Bean and Kale Soup

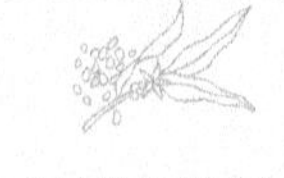 

PREP TIME
20 MINUTES

COOK TIME
30 MINUTES

INGREDIENTS :

- 2 tbsp olive oil
- 1 onion, diced
- 3 garlic cloves, minced
- 2 carrots, peeled and sliced
- 2 celery stalks, sliced
- 2 (15 oz) cans no-salt-added white beans, rinsed and drained
- 6 cups low-sodium chicken or vegetable broth
- 2 cups chopped kale, stems removed
- 1 tsp dried thyme
- 1/2 tsp dried rosemary
- Salt and pepper to taste
- Grated Parmesan cheese for serving (optional)

PROCEDURE :

1. In a large pot or Dutch oven, heat the olive oil over medium heat. Add the onion and cook for 3-4 minutes until translucent.

2. Stir in the garlic, carrots, and celery. Cook for 5 minutes, stirring occasionally, until the vegetables start to soften.

3. Add the white beans, broth, kale, thyme, and rosemary. Season with salt and pepper.

4. Bring the soup to a boil, then reduce heat and let it simmer for 20-25 minutes, until the vegetables are tender.

5. Use an immersion blender to puree about half of the soup, leaving some texture. Alternatively, you can transfer 2-3 cups of the soup to a regular blender and blend until smooth, then return it to the pot.

6. Taste and adjust seasoning as needed.

7. Ladle the white bean and kale soup into bowls. Top with a sprinkle of grated Parmesan cheese if desired.

This hearty, nutrient-dense soup is packed with fiber, protein, and vitamins from the white beans and kale. It makes a satisfying and comforting meal. You can customize it by adding other vegetables like spinach, zucchini, or potatoes.

80. Chicken Tortilla Soup

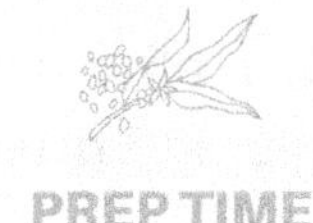

PREP TIME
20 MINUTES

COOK TIME
30 MINUTES

INGREDIENTS :

- 1 lb boneless, skinless chicken breasts, cut into 1-inch pieces
- 1 tbsp olive oil
- 1 onion, diced
- 3 garlic cloves, minced
- 2 tsp ground cumin
- 1 tsp chili powder
- 1 (15 oz) can no-salt-added diced tomatoes
- 4 cups low-sodium chicken broth
- 1 (15 oz) can no-salt-added black beans, rinsed and drained
- 1 cup frozen corn
- 2 cups shredded cabbage or kale
- Juice of 1 lime
- Salt and pepper to taste
- Baked tortilla strips or crushed baked tortilla chips for serving
- Chopped avocado, cilantro, and plain Greek yogurt for garnish (optional)

PROCEDURE :

1. In a large pot or Dutch oven, heat the olive oil over medium-high heat. Add the chicken and cook for 3-4 minutes, until lightly browned.

2. Add the onion and garlic and cook for 2-3 minutes until fragrant.

3. Stir in the cumin, chili powder, diced tomatoes, chicken broth, black beans, and corn. Bring the soup to a boil.

4. Reduce heat and let the soup simmer for 15-20 minutes, until the chicken is cooked through.

5. Stir in the shredded cabbage/kale and lime juice. Season with salt and pepper to taste.

6. Serve the chicken tortilla soup hot, topped with baked tortilla strips or crushed baked tortilla chips. Add avocado, cilantro, and a dollop of Greek yogurt if desired.

This chicken tortilla soup is packed with protein, fiber, and vegetables, making it a great option for managing type 2 diabetes. The cabbage or kale adds extra nutrients while the lime juice and spices provide flavor without added sugar.

81. Grilled Salmon with Asparagus

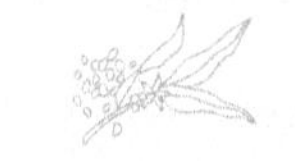

PREP TIME
20 MINUTES

COOK TIME
30 MINUTES

INGREDIENTS:

- 4 (6 oz) salmon fillets
- 2 tbsp olive oil, divided
- 1 tsp lemon zest
- 1 tbsp lemon juice
- 1 tsp Dijon mustard
- 1 tsp dried dill
- Salt and pepper to taste
- 1 lb asparagus, trimmed
- 1 tbsp balsamic vinegar

PROCEDURE:

1. Preheat grill or grill pan to medium-high heat.

2. In a small bowl, whisk together 1 tbsp olive oil, lemon zest, lemon juice, Dijon mustard, and dried dill. Season with salt and pepper.

3. Place the salmon fillets in a shallow dish and pour the lemon-dill marinade over the top. Let marinate for 15-20 minutes.

4. In a large bowl, toss the asparagus with the remaining 1 tbsp olive oil and season with salt and pepper.

5. Grill the salmon for 4-5 minutes per side, until opaque and cooked through. Grill the asparagus for 5-7 minutes, turning occasionally, until tender-crisp.

6. Transfer the grilled salmon and asparagus to a serving platter. Drizzle the asparagus with the balsamic vinegar.

7. Serve the grilled salmon and asparagus immediately.

This grilled salmon and asparagus dish is an excellent choice for managing type 2 diabetes. Salmon is high in protein and healthy omega-3 fatty acids, while asparagus is low in carbs and high in fiber. The simple lemon-dill marinade and balsamic drizzle add flavor without added sugar.

82. Baked Chicken with Brussels Sprouts

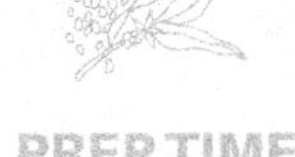

PREP TIME
20 MINUTES

COOK TIME
30 MINUTES

INGREDIENTS:

- 1 lb boneless, skinless chicken breasts, cut into 1-inch pieces
- 1 lb Brussels sprouts, trimmed and halved
- 2 tbsp olive oil, divided
- 1 tsp dried thyme
- 1 tsp garlic powder
- Salt and pepper to taste
- 2 tbsp grated Parmesan cheese (optional)
- Lemon wedges for serving

PROCEDURE:

1. Preheat oven to 400°F. Line a large baking sheet with parchment paper.

2. In a large bowl, toss the chicken pieces with 1 tbsp of the olive oil, thyme, garlic powder, and a pinch of salt and pepper.

3. In a separate bowl, toss the Brussels sprouts with the remaining 1 tbsp olive oil and season with salt and pepper.

4. Spread the chicken and Brussels sprouts in a single layer on the prepared baking sheet.

5. Bake for 20-25 minutes, stirring halfway, until the chicken is cooked through and the Brussels sprouts are tender and lightly browned.

6. Remove from oven and sprinkle the Parmesan cheese over the top, if using.

7. Serve the baked chicken and Brussels sprouts immediately, with lemon wedges on the side.

This simple one-pan meal is perfect for managing type 2 diabetes. The lean protein from the chicken and the fiber-rich Brussels sprouts make it a nutritious and balanced dish. The Parmesan cheese adds a nice flavor boost without significantly increasing the carb content.

You can customize this recipe by using different herbs and spices or adding other roasted vegetables like sweet potatoes or cauliflower.

83. Beef Stir-Fry with Vegetables

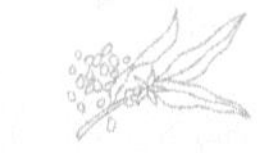

PREP TIME
20 MINUTES

COOK TIME
30 MINUTES

INGREDIENTS :

- 1 lb lean beef sirloin or flank steak, thinly sliced
- 2 tbsp low-sodium soy sauce
- 1 tbsp rice vinegar
- 1 tsp sesame oil
- 1 tbsp cornstarch
- 2 tbsp olive oil, divided
- 3 garlic cloves, minced
- 1 tbsp grated fresh ginger
- 1 red bell pepper, sliced
- 1 cup broccoli florets
- 1 cup sliced mushrooms
- 1 cup snow peas or snap peas
- 2 cups cooked brown rice

For the Sauce:
- 2 tbsp low-sodium soy sauce
- 1 tbsp rice vinegar
- 1 tsp sesame oil
- 1 tsp honey
- 1 tsp cornstarch

PROCEDURE :

1. In a medium bowl, combine the sliced beef, 2 tbsp soy sauce, 1 tbsp rice vinegar, 1 tsp sesame oil, and 1 tbsp cornstarch. Toss to coat the beef and let marinate for 15 minutes.

2. In a small bowl, whisk together the sauce ingredients (2 tbsp soy sauce, 1 tbsp rice vinegar, 1 tsp sesame oil, 1 tsp honey, 1 tsp cornstarch).

3. Heat 1 tbsp olive oil in a large skillet or wok over high heat. Add the beef and stir-fry for 2-3 minutes until browned. Remove the beef from the pan and set aside.

4. Add the remaining 1 tbsp olive oil to the pan. Stir in the garlic and ginger and cook for 1 minute until fragrant.

5. Add the bell pepper, broccoli, mushrooms, and snow peas. Stir-fry for 3-4 minutes until the vegetables are crisp-tender.

6. Return the beef to the pan and pour in the sauce. Bring to a simmer and cook for 2-3 minutes, stirring frequently, until the sauce has thickened.

7. Serve the beef and vegetable stir-fry over the cooked brown rice.

This beef stir-fry is packed with lean protein, fiber-rich vegetables, and complex carbs from the brown rice. The balanced macronutrients make it an excellent choice for managing type 2 diabetes.

84. Turkey Meatballs with Zoodles

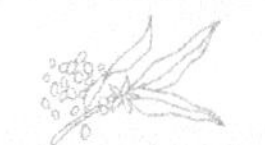 

PREP TIME
20 MINUTES

COOK TIME
30 MINUTES

INGREDIENTS :

For the Meatballs:
- 1 lb ground turkey
- 1/2 cup whole wheat breadcrumbs
- 1 egg, lightly beaten
- 2 tbsp grated Parmesan cheese
- 2 garlic cloves, minced
- 1 tsp dried oregano
- 1/2 tsp salt
- 1/4 tsp black pepper

For the Zoodles:
- 3 medium zucchini, spiralized into noodles
- 2 tbsp olive oil
- 2 garlic cloves, minced
- 1 (14.5 oz) can no-salt-added diced tomatoes
- 1/4 cup fresh basil leaves, chopped
- Salt and pepper to taste

PROCEDURE :

1. Preheat oven to 400°F. Line a baking sheet with parchment paper.

2. In a large bowl, combine all the meatball ingredients and mix well. Roll the mixture into 1-inch meatballs and place them on the prepared baking sheet.

3. Bake the meatballs for 18-20 minutes, until cooked through.

4. While the meatballs are baking, heat the olive oil in a large skillet over medium heat. Add the garlic and cook for 1 minute until fragrant.

5. Add the spiralized zucchini noodles to the skillet and sauté for 3-5 minutes, until the zoodles are tender but still have some bite.

6. Stir in the diced tomatoes and their juices. Cook for 2-3 minutes more, until heated through.

7. Remove the skillet from heat and stir in the chopped basil. Season with salt and pepper to taste.

8. Serve the turkey meatballs over the zucchini noodles.

This dish is a great way to enjoy lean protein, vegetables, and whole grains. The turkey meatballs are flavorful and the zoodles provide a low-carb alternative to pasta. It's a healthy and satisfying meal.

85. Pork Tenderloin with Green Beans

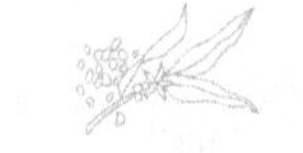

PREP TIME
20 MINUTES

COOK TIME
30 MINUTES

INGREDIENTS:

- 1 lb pork tenderloin, trimmed of excess fat
- 2 tbsp olive oil, divided
- 1 tsp garlic powder
- 1 tsp dried thyme
- Salt and pepper to taste
- 1 lb green beans, trimmed
- 2 cloves garlic, minced
- 2 tbsp low-sodium soy sauce
- 1 tbsp lemon juice
- 1 tsp Dijon mustard

PROCEDURE:

1. Preheat oven to 400°F. Line a baking sheet with foil or parchment paper.

2. In a small bowl, combine 1 tbsp olive oil, garlic powder, thyme, and a pinch of salt and pepper. Rub this mixture all over the pork tenderloin.

3. Place the pork tenderloin on the prepared baking sheet. Roast for 20-25 minutes, until the internal temperature reaches 145°F. Let rest for 5 minutes before slicing.

4. While the pork is roasting, heat the remaining 1 tbsp olive oil in a large skillet over medium-high heat. Add the green beans and sauté for 5-7 minutes, until crisp-tender.

5. Add the minced garlic to the skillet and cook for 1 minute until fragrant.

6. In a small bowl, whisk together the soy sauce, lemon juice, and Dijon mustard. Pour this sauce over the green beans and toss to coat.

7. Serve the sliced pork tenderloin with the sautéed garlic-soy green beans on the side.

This pork tenderloin and green bean dish is a simple, healthy, and delicious meal. The lean pork provides protein, while the green beans add fiber and vitamins. The flavorful soy-lemon sauce complements the vegetables perfectly.

You can adjust the cooking time for the pork based on the thickness of the tenderloin. Serve with roasted potatoes or a side salad for a complete meal.

86. Stuffed Bell Peppers with Ground Turkey

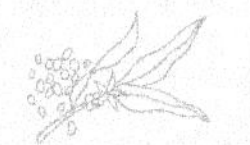

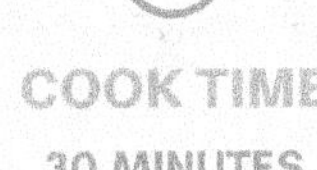

PREP TIME
20 MINUTES

COOK TIME
30 MINUTES

INGREDIENTS:

- 6 bell peppers (any color), halved lengthwise and seeds/membranes removed
- 1 lb ground turkey
- 1 cup cooked brown rice
- 1 (14.5 oz) can no-salt-added diced tomatoes
- 1/2 cup diced onion
- 2 garlic cloves, minced
- 1 tsp dried oregano
- 1/2 tsp ground cumin
- 1/4 tsp cayenne pepper (optional)
- Salt and pepper to taste
- 1/2 cup shredded low-fat mozzarella cheese (optional)

PROCEDURE:

1. Preheat oven to 375°F. Arrange the bell pepper halves in a baking dish or on a rimmed baking sheet.

2. In a large skillet over medium heat, cook the ground turkey, breaking it up with a wooden spoon, until no longer pink, about 5-7 minutes.

3. Drain any excess fat from the skillet. Add the cooked brown rice, diced tomatoes, onion, garlic, oregano, cumin, and cayenne (if using). Season with salt and pepper.

4. Spoon the turkey-rice mixture evenly into the bell pepper halves.

5. Cover the baking dish or sheet with foil and bake for 25-30 minutes, until the peppers are tender.

6. Remove the foil and sprinkle the tops of the stuffed peppers with the shredded mozzarella cheese, if using.

7. Return the dish to the oven and bake for 5-10 more minutes, until the cheese is melted.

8. Serve the stuffed bell peppers hot.

These stuffed bell peppers are a delicious and healthy meal. The ground turkey provides lean protein, while the brown rice and peppers offer fiber and complex carbs. This dish is perfect for managing type 2 diabetes.

You can customize the filling by adding more vegetables or using different herbs and spices. Enjoy!

87. Grilled Shrimp with Quinoa

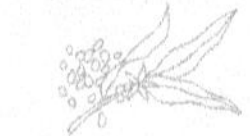

PREP TIME
20 MINUTES

COOK TIME
30 MINUTES

INGREDIENTS :

- 1 lb large shrimp, peeled and deveined
- 2 tbsp olive oil
- 2 tsp lemon juice
- 1 tsp paprika
- 1/2 tsp garlic powder
- 1/4 tsp cayenne pepper (optional)
- Salt and pepper to taste
- 1 cup uncooked quinoa, rinsed
- 2 cups low-sodium chicken or vegetable broth
- 1 cup cherry tomatoes, halved
- 1/2 cup diced cucumber
- 2 tbsp chopped fresh parsley
- 1 tbsp lemon zest
- 2 tbsp crumbled feta cheese (optional)

PROCEDURE :

1. In a large bowl, toss the shrimp with 1 tbsp of the olive oil, lemon juice, paprika, garlic powder, and cayenne (if using). Season with salt and pepper. Cover and refrigerate for 30 minutes.

2. In a medium saucepan, combine the quinoa and broth. Bring to a boil, then reduce heat, cover, and simmer for 15-20 minutes, until the quinoa is tender and the liquid is absorbed. Fluff with a fork and let cool slightly.

3. Preheat grill or grill pan to medium-high heat. Thread the marinated shrimp onto skewers.

4. Grill the shrimp for 2-3 minutes per side, until opaque and cooked through.

5. In a large bowl, combine the cooked quinoa, tomatoes, cucumber, parsley, and lemon zest. Drizzle with the remaining 1 tbsp olive oil and toss to coat.

6. Serve the grilled shrimp over the quinoa salad. Top with crumbled feta cheese if desired.

This grilled shrimp and quinoa dish is high in protein, fiber, and healthy fats, making it an excellent choice for managing type 2 diabetes. The quinoa provides complex carbs while the shrimp and vegetables keep the carb content low.

88. Vegetable Stir-Fry with Tofu

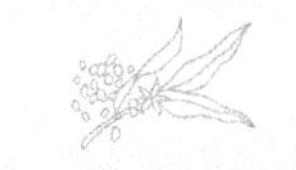

PREP TIME
20 MINUTES

COOK TIME
30 MINUTES

INGREDIENTS:

- 1 block (14 oz) extra-firm tofu, drained and cubed
- 2 tbsp low-sodium soy sauce, divided
- 1 tbsp sesame oil, divided
- 2 tbsp olive oil, divided
- 1 red bell pepper, sliced
- 1 cup broccoli florets
- 1 cup sliced mushrooms
- 1 cup snow peas or snap peas
- 3 garlic cloves, minced
- 1 tbsp grated fresh ginger
- 1 tsp rice vinegar
- 1 tsp sesame seeds (optional)
- Salt and pepper to taste
- Cooked brown rice, for serving (optional)

PROCEDURE:

1. In a medium bowl, toss the cubed tofu with 1 tbsp soy sauce and 1 tsp sesame oil. Let marinate for 10-15 minutes.

2. Heat 1 tbsp olive oil in a large skillet or wok over medium-high heat. Add the marinated tofu and cook for 5-7 minutes, turning occasionally, until lightly browned. Remove tofu from the pan and set aside.

3. Add the remaining 1 tbsp olive oil to the pan. Stir-fry the bell pepper, broccoli, mushrooms, and snow/snap peas for 5-7 minutes, until crisp-tender.

4. Push the vegetables to the side of the pan. Add the garlic and ginger to the center and cook for 1 minute until fragrant.

5. Add the cooked tofu back to the pan. Drizzle with the remaining 1 tbsp soy sauce, 2 tsp sesame oil, and rice vinegar. Toss everything together until well combined.

6. Remove from heat and sprinkle with sesame seeds, if using. Season with salt and pepper to taste.

7. Serve the vegetable stir-fry over cooked brown rice, if desired.

This vegetable stir-fry with tofu is a great option for managing type 2 diabetes. Tofu provides plant-based protein, while the variety of vegetables add fiber, vitamins, and minerals without many carbs. The simple soy-sesame sauce adds flavor without added sugar.

89. Baked Cod with Cauliflower Rice

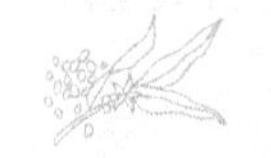

PREP TIME
20 MINUTES

COOK TIME
30 MINUTES

INGREDIENTS :

- 4 (6 oz) cod fillets
- 2 tbsp olive oil, divided
- 1 tsp paprika
- 1 tsp garlic powder
- Salt and pepper to taste
- 1 head of cauliflower, riced (about 4 cups riced cauliflower)
- 1 onion, diced
- 2 garlic cloves, minced
- 1 cup diced tomatoes
- 2 tbsp chopped fresh parsley
- Lemon wedges for serving

PROCEDURE :

1. Preheat oven to 400°F. Line a baking sheet with parchment paper.

2. Place the cod fillets on the prepared baking sheet. Drizzle with 1 tbsp of the olive oil and sprinkle with the paprika, garlic powder, salt, and pepper.

3. Bake the cod for 12-15 minutes, until it flakes easily with a fork.

4. While the cod is baking, heat the remaining 1 tbsp olive oil in a large skillet over medium heat. Add the riced cauliflower, onion, and garlic. Sauté for 5-7 minutes, until the cauliflower is tender.

5. Stir in the diced tomatoes and chopped parsley. Season with salt and pepper.

6. Serve the baked cod fillets over the cauliflower rice. Garnish with lemon wedges.

This baked cod and cauliflower rice dish is an excellent choice for managing type 2 diabetes. Cod is a lean, high-protein fish that is low in carbs. The cauliflower rice provides a low-carb alternative to traditional rice.

The simple seasoning on the cod and the fresh tomato-parsley mixture add lots of flavor without the need for heavy sauces. This makes a well-balanced, nutrient-dense meal.

90. Chicken Fajitas with Peppers and Onions

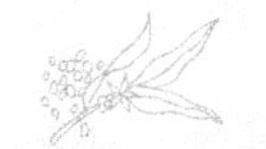

PREP TIME
20 MINUTES

COOK TIME
30 MINUTES

INGREDIENTS :

- 1 lb boneless, skinless chicken breasts, sliced into strips
- 1 red bell pepper, sliced into strips
- 1 green bell pepper, sliced into strips
- 1 onion, sliced into strips
- 2 tbsp olive oil
- 1 tsp chili powder
- 1 tsp cumin
- 1/2 tsp garlic powder
- 1/4 tsp cayenne pepper (optional)
- Salt and pepper to taste
- 8 small whole wheat tortillas

PROCEDURE :

1. In a large skillet or wok, heat the olive oil over medium-high heat.

2. Add the chicken strips and season with chili powder, cumin, garlic powder, cayenne (if using), salt, and pepper. Cook for 5-7 minutes, stirring occasionally, until the chicken is cooked through.

3. Add the sliced bell peppers and onions to the skillet. Cook for an additional 5-7 minutes, stirring frequently, until the vegetables are tender-crisp.

4. Serve the chicken and vegetable mixture in the whole wheat tortillas. Top with your desired toppings such as avocado, salsa, low-fat sour cream, or shredded cheese.

This recipe is diabetes-friendly as it uses lean protein (chicken), plenty of fiber-rich vegetables, and whole wheat tortillas. The spices add flavor without the need for added sugars or high-sodium sauces. Portion control is also important, so stick to 1-2 fajitas per serving.

91. Baked Halibut with Mixed Vegetables

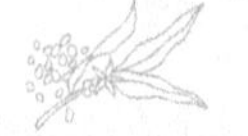 

PREP TIME
20 MINUTES

COOK TIME
30 MINUTES

INGREDIENTS :

- 4 (6 oz) halibut fillets
- 2 tbsp olive oil, divided
- 1 tsp lemon zest
- 1 tbsp lemon juice
- 1 tsp dried dill
- Salt and pepper to taste
- 1 cup broccoli florets
- 1 cup sliced zucchini
- 1 cup sliced yellow squash
- 1 cup cherry tomatoes, halved
- 2 garlic cloves, minced
- 1 tbsp chopped fresh parsley

PROCEDURE :

1. Preheat oven to 400°F. Line a baking sheet with parchment paper.

2. In a small bowl, combine 1 tbsp olive oil, lemon zest, lemon juice, and dried dill. Season with salt and pepper.

3. Place the halibut fillets on the prepared baking sheet. Brush the tops of the fish with the lemon-dill mixture.

4. In a large bowl, toss the broccoli, zucchini, yellow squash, and cherry tomatoes with the remaining 1 tbsp olive oil. Season with salt and pepper.

5. Arrange the seasoned vegetables around the halibut fillets on the baking sheet.

6. Bake for 15-18 minutes, until the fish is opaque and flakes easily with a fork and the vegetables are tender.

7. Remove the baking sheet from the oven and sprinkle the minced garlic and chopped parsley over the vegetables.

8. Serve the baked halibut immediately, with the roasted vegetables on the side.

This baked halibut and vegetable dish is an excellent choice for managing type 2 diabetes. Halibut is a lean, high-protein fish that is low in carbs. The mixed vegetables provide fiber, vitamins, and minerals without adding many carbs.

The simple lemon-dill seasoning adds flavor without the need for heavy sauces or dressings. This makes a well-balanced, nutrient-dense meal.

92. Turkey and Vegetable Stuffed Zucchini Boats

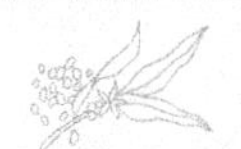 

PREP TIME
20 MINUTES

COOK TIME
30 MINUTES

INGREDIENTS :

- 4 medium zucchini, halved lengthwise
- 1 lb ground turkey
- 1 onion, diced
- 2 garlic cloves, minced
- 1 cup diced bell pepper
- 1 cup diced mushrooms
- 1 (14.5 oz) can no-salt-added diced tomatoes
- 1 tsp dried oregano
- 1/2 tsp dried basil
- Salt and pepper to taste
- 1/2 cup shredded low-fat mozzarella cheese (optional)

PROCEDURE :

1. Preheat oven to 375°F. Scoop out the seeds and flesh from the center of each zucchini half, leaving a 1/4-inch shell. Chop the scooped out zucchini flesh.

2. In a large skillet over medium heat, cook the ground turkey, breaking it up with a wooden spoon, until no longer pink, about 5-7 minutes.

3. Add the diced onion, garlic, bell pepper, mushrooms, and chopped zucchini flesh to the skillet. Cook for 5-7 minutes, until the vegetables are tender.

4. Stir in the diced tomatoes, oregano, and basil. Season with salt and pepper.

5. Arrange the zucchini boats in a baking dish. Spoon the turkey-vegetable mixture evenly into the zucchini boats.

6. If using, sprinkle the tops of the stuffed zucchini boats with the shredded mozzarella cheese.

7. Bake for 20-25 minutes, until the zucchini is tender and the cheese is melted.

8. Serve the stuffed zucchini boats hot.

These turkey and vegetable stuffed zucchini boats are a great low-carb, high-protein option for managing type 2 diabetes. The zucchini provides fiber, while the turkey and vegetables offer a nutrient-dense filling. The cheese is optional, but adds a nice creamy texture.

You can customize the filling by using different herbs, spices, or additional vegetables. This makes a satisfying and healthy main dish.

93. Lemon Herb Chicken with Broccoli

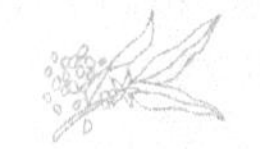 

PREP TIME
20 MINUTES

COOK TIME
30 MINUTES

INGREDIENTS:

- 1 lb boneless, skinless chicken breasts
- 2 tbsp olive oil
- 2 tbsp lemon juice
- 1 tsp dried oregano
- 1 tsp dried basil
- 1 tsp garlic powder
- Salt and pepper to taste
- 4 cups broccoli florets

PROCEDURE:

1. Preheat oven to 400°F.

2. In a small bowl, combine the olive oil, lemon juice, oregano, basil, garlic powder, salt, and pepper.

3. Place the chicken breasts in a baking dish and pour the lemon herb mixture over the top, making sure to coat the chicken evenly.

4. Bake the chicken for 20-25 minutes, or until it reaches an internal temperature of 165°F.

5. During the last 10 minutes of baking, add the broccoli florets to the baking dish. Toss the broccoli with the remaining lemon herb sauce.

6. Serve the lemon herb chicken with the roasted broccoli.

This recipe is diabetes-friendly for a few reasons:

- Chicken is a lean protein that is low in carbs and high in protein, which helps regulate blood sugar levels.
- Broccoli is a non-starchy vegetable that is high in fiber, vitamins, and minerals.
- The lemon and herb seasoning adds flavor without the need for added sugars or high-sodium sauces.
- Baking the chicken and broccoli together keeps the dish simple and easy to prepare.

Portion control is still important, so aim for a 4-6 oz serving of chicken and 1 cup of broccoli per serving.

94. Spaghetti Squash with Meatballs 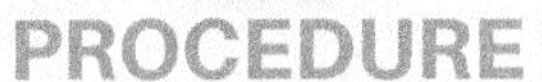

PREP TIME
20 MINUTES

COOK TIME
30 MINUTES

INGREDIENTS:

For the Meatballs:
- 1 lb ground turkey or lean ground beef
- 1/4 cup whole wheat breadcrumbs
- 1 egg, lightly beaten
- 2 tbsp grated Parmesan cheese
- 2 garlic cloves, minced
- 1 tsp dried oregano
- 1/2 tsp salt
- 1/4 tsp black pepper

For the Spaghetti Squash and Marinara:
- 1 medium spaghetti squash, halved lengthwise and seeds removed
- 1 tbsp olive oil
- 1 (24 oz) jar no-sugar-added marinara sauce
- 2 cups baby spinach (optional)
- Grated Parmesan cheese for serving (optional)

PROCEDURE:

1. Preheat oven to 400°F. Line a baking sheet with parchment paper.

2. Make the meatballs: In a large bowl, combine all the meatball ingredients and mix well. Roll the mixture into 1-inch meatballs and place them on the prepared baking sheet.

3. Bake the meatballs for 18-20 minutes, until cooked through.

4. While the meatballs are baking, place the spaghetti squash halves cut-side down on the baking sheet. Bake for 35-45 minutes, until tender when pierced with a fork.

5. Remove the spaghetti squash and meatballs from the oven. Let the squash cool for 5 minutes, then use a fork to shred the flesh into spaghetti-like strands.

6. In a large skillet, heat the olive oil over medium heat. Add the shredded spaghetti squash and sauté for 2-3 minutes.

7. Pour in the marinara sauce and stir to coat the squash. Add the baby spinach (if using) and cook for 2-3 more minutes until the spinach is wilted.

8. Serve the spaghetti squash and marinara topped with the baked turkey meatballs. Sprinkle with grated Parmesan cheese if desired.

This dish is a great option for managing type 2 diabetes. The spaghetti squash provides a low-carb alternative to pasta, while the turkey meatballs offer lean protein. The marinara sauce adds flavor without added sugar.

95. Grilled Pork Chops with Apple Slaw

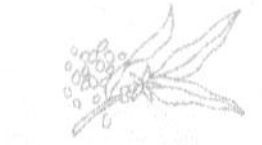 

PREP TIME
20 MINUTES

COOK TIME
30 MINUTES

INGREDIENTS :

For the Pork Chops:
- 4 (6 oz) boneless pork chops
- 1 tbsp olive oil
- 1 tsp garlic powder
- 1 tsp dried thyme
- Salt and pepper to taste

For the Apple Slaw:
- 2 cups shredded green cabbage
- 1 cup shredded red cabbage
- 1 Granny Smith apple, julienned
- 1/4 cup plain Greek yogurt
- 1 tbsp apple cider vinegar
- 1 tsp Dijon mustard
- 1 tsp honey
- Salt and pepper to taste

PROCEDURE :

1. Preheat your grill or grill pan to medium-high heat.

2. In a small bowl, combine the olive oil, garlic powder, thyme, salt, and pepper. Rub this mixture all over the pork chops.

3. Grill the pork chops for 4-5 minutes per side, or until they reach an internal temperature of 145°F. Transfer to a plate and let rest for 5 minutes.

4. In a large bowl, combine the shredded green and red cabbage, julienned apple, Greek yogurt, apple cider vinegar, Dijon mustard, honey, salt, and pepper. Toss to coat the slaw.

5. Serve the grilled pork chops with the apple slaw on the side.

This dish is a great option for managing type 2 diabetes for the following reasons:

- Pork chops are a lean protein that is low in carbs and high in protein.
- The apple slaw provides a crunchy, fiber-rich topping without added sugars.
- Grilling the pork chops keeps the dish light and healthy.
- The combination of protein, fiber, and healthy fats helps regulate blood sugar levels.

Portion control is still important, so aim for a 4-6 oz serving of pork chops and 1 cup of apple slaw per person. Serve with a side of roasted vegetables or a small serving of whole grains for a complete, diabetes-friendly meal.

96. Cauliflower Crust Pizza with Veggies

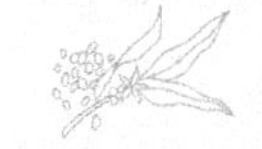 

PREP TIME
20 MINUTES

COOK TIME
30 MINUTES

INGREDIENTS :

For the Cauliflower Crust:
- 1 head of cauliflower, riced (about 4 cups riced cauliflower)
- 1 egg, beaten
- 1/2 cup shredded part-skim mozzarella cheese
- 2 tbsp grated Parmesan cheese
- 1 tsp dried oregano
- 1/2 tsp garlic powder
- 1/4 tsp salt

For the Toppings:
- 1/2 cup marinara sauce
- 1 cup shredded part-skim mozzarella cheese
- 1 cup mixed vegetables (such as sliced bell peppers, onions, mushrooms, spinach)

PROCEDURE :

1. Preheat your oven to 400°F. Line a baking sheet with parchment paper.

2. To make the cauliflower crust, place the riced cauliflower in a microwave-safe bowl and microwave for 5-7 minutes, until tender. Allow to cool slightly.

3. Transfer the cooked cauliflower to a clean kitchen towel or cheesecloth and squeeze out as much moisture as possible.

4. In a medium bowl, combine the squeezed cauliflower, beaten egg, mozzarella, Parmesan, oregano, garlic powder, and salt. Mix well.

5. Press the cauliflower mixture onto the prepared baking sheet, forming a thin, even crust. Bake the crust for 20-25 minutes, until golden brown.

7. Remove the crust from the oven and top with the marinara sauce, shredded mozzarella, and your choice of vegetables.

8. Return the pizza to the oven and bake for an additional 10-15 minutes, until the cheese is melted and bubbly. Slice and serve the cauliflower crust pizza immediately.

This cauliflower crust pizza is a great option for managing type 2 diabetes because:

- Cauliflower is a low-carb, high-fiber vegetable that replaces the traditional wheat-based crust.
- The toppings are all non-starchy vegetables, which are high in fiber, vitamins, and minerals.
- The cheese provides protein and healthy fats without added sugars.
- Portion control is important, so aim for 1-2 slices per serving.

97. Beef and Broccoli Stir-Fry

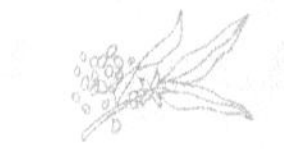

PREP TIME
20 MINUTES

COOK TIME
30 MINUTES

INGREDIENTS:

- 1 lb flank steak, thinly sliced
- 2 tbsp low-sodium soy sauce
- 1 tbsp rice vinegar
- 1 tsp sesame oil
- 1 tsp grated ginger
- 2 cloves garlic, minced
- 2 tbsp olive oil
- 4 cups broccoli florets
- 1 red bell pepper, sliced
- 1 onion, sliced
- Salt and pepper to taste

PROCEDURE:

1. In a medium bowl, combine the sliced beef, soy sauce, rice vinegar, sesame oil, ginger, and garlic. Toss to coat the beef and let marinate for 15-20 minutes.

2. Heat the olive oil in a large skillet or wok over high heat.

3. Add the marinated beef and stir-fry for 2-3 minutes, until the beef is lightly browned. Remove the beef from the pan and set aside.

4. Add the broccoli, bell pepper, and onion to the pan. Stir-fry for 4-5 minutes, until the vegetables are tender-crisp.

5. Return the beef to the pan and toss everything together. Season with salt and pepper to taste.

6. Serve the beef and broccoli stir-fry immediately, over a bed of steamed brown rice or cauliflower rice.

This recipe is diabetes-friendly for the following reasons:

- Flank steak is a lean protein that is low in carbs and high in protein.
- Broccoli, bell peppers, and onions are non-starchy vegetables that are high in fiber, vitamins, and minerals.
- The soy sauce, rice vinegar, and sesame oil provide flavor without the need for added sugars.
- Stir-frying the ingredients keeps the dish light and healthy.

Portion control is still important, so aim for a 4-6 oz serving of the beef and broccoli mixture, along with a small serving of brown rice or cauliflower rice.

98. Grilled Swordfish with Mango Salsa

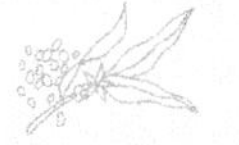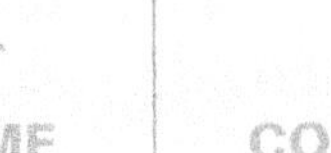

PREP TIME
20 MINUTES

COOK TIME
30 MINUTES

INGREDIENTS:

For the Mango Salsa:
- 1 ripe mango, diced
- 1/2 red onion, finely chopped
- 1 jalapeño, seeded and finely chopped
- 1/4 cup chopped fresh cilantro
- 2 tbsp lime juice
- 1 tsp olive oil
- Salt and pepper to taste

For the Swordfish:
- 4 (6 oz) swordfish steaks
- 1 tbsp olive oil
- 1 tsp chili powder
- 1 tsp garlic powder
- Salt and pepper to taste

PROCEDURE:

1. Make the mango salsa: In a medium bowl, combine the diced mango, red onion, jalapeño, cilantro, lime juice, and olive oil. Season with salt and pepper to taste. Cover and refrigerate until ready to serve.

2. Preheat your grill or grill pan to medium-high heat.

3. Pat the swordfish steaks dry and brush them with the 1 tbsp of olive oil. Season both sides with the chili powder, garlic powder, salt, and pepper.

4. Grill the swordfish for 3-4 minutes per side, or until it flakes easily with a fork and reaches an internal temperature of 145°F.

5. Serve the grilled swordfish immediately, topped with the chilled mango salsa.

This dish is a great option for managing type 2 diabetes for the following reasons:

- Swordfish is a lean, high-protein seafood that is low in carbs.
- The mango salsa provides a sweet and tangy topping without added sugars.
- Grilling the swordfish keeps the dish light and healthy.
- The combination of protein, healthy fats, and fiber-rich vegetables helps regulate blood sugar levels.

Portion control is still important, so aim for a 4-6 oz serving of swordfish and 1/2 cup of mango salsa per person. Serve with a side of roasted vegetables or a fresh salad for a complete, diabetes-friendly meal.

99. Eggplant Parmesan (baked, not fried)

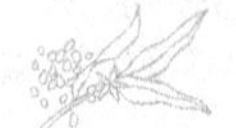 

PREP TIME
20 MINUTES

COOK TIME
30 MINUTES

INGREDIENTS :

- 2 medium eggplants, sliced into 1/4-inch thick rounds
- 1 cup whole wheat breadcrumbs
- 1/2 cup grated Parmesan cheese
- 2 tsp dried oregano
- 1 tsp garlic powder
- 1/4 tsp red pepper flakes (optional)
- 2 eggs, beaten
- 1 cup marinara sauce
- 1 cup shredded part-skim mozzarella cheese

PROCEDURE :

1. Preheat oven to 375°F. Line a baking sheet with parchment paper.

2. In a shallow bowl, combine the breadcrumbs, Parmesan, oregano, garlic powder, and red pepper flakes (if using).

3. Dip the eggplant slices into the beaten eggs, then coat them in the breadcrumb mixture, pressing gently to adhere. Arrange the breaded eggplant slices in a single layer on the prepared baking sheet.

5. Bake for 20 minutes, flip the slices, and bake for an additional 15-20 minutes, until the eggplant is tender and the breading is golden brown.

6. Spread 1/2 cup of the marinara sauce in the bottom of a 9x13 inch baking dish. Arrange the baked eggplant slices in a single layer over the sauce.

7. Top the eggplant with the remaining 1/2 cup of marinara sauce and the shredded mozzarella cheese.

8. Bake for an additional 15-20 minutes, until the cheese is melted and bubbly. Let the eggplant parmesan cool for 5 minutes before serving.

This baked eggplant parmesan is a diabetes-friendly version of the classic dish. The key features that make it suitable for managing type 2 diabetes are:

- Eggplant is a low-carb, high-fiber vegetable.
- Whole wheat breadcrumbs and Parmesan provide a crunchy coating without added sugars.
- Baking instead of frying reduces the amount of fat and calories.

100. Turkey and Spinach Stuffed Portobello Mushrooms

PREP TIME
20 MINUTES

COOK TIME
30 MINUTES

INGREDIENTS:

- 4 large portobello mushroom caps, stems removed and chopped
- 1 lb ground turkey
- 2 cups fresh spinach, chopped
- 1/2 cup diced onion
- 2 cloves garlic, minced
- 1 tsp dried oregano
- 1/4 tsp red pepper flakes (optional)
- 1/2 cup shredded part-skim mozzarella cheese
- Salt and pepper to taste

PROCEDURE:

1. Preheat your oven to 400°F. Lightly grease a baking sheet or oven-safe dish.

2. Place the portobello mushroom caps, gill-side up, on the prepared baking sheet.

3. In a large skillet over medium heat, cook the ground turkey, chopped mushroom stems, onion, and garlic until the turkey is browned and the vegetables are tender, about 5-7 minutes. Drain any excess fat.

4. Add the chopped spinach, oregano, and red pepper flakes (if using) to the skillet. Cook for an additional 2-3 minutes, until the spinach is wilted.

5. Spoon the turkey and spinach mixture evenly into the portobello mushroom caps. Top each cap with 2 tbsp of shredded mozzarella cheese.

6. Bake the stuffed mushrooms for 15-20 minutes, until the mushrooms are tender and the cheese is melted and bubbly. Serve the stuffed portobello mushrooms immediately.

This dish is a great option for managing type 2 diabetes for the following reasons:

- Portobello mushrooms are a low-carb, high-fiber vegetable that serve as the "base" for the dish.
- Ground turkey is a lean protein that is low in carbs and high in protein.
- Spinach is a nutrient-dense, non-starchy vegetable that provides fiber, vitamins, and minerals.
- The small amount of mozzarella cheese provides healthy fats without added sugars.
- Baking the stuffed mushrooms keeps the dish light and healthy.

101. Lamb Chops with Mint Yogurt Sauce

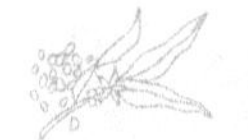

PREP TIME
20 MINUTES

COOK TIME
30 MINUTES

INGREDIENTS:

- 8 lamb chops (about 1.5 lbs)
- 2 tbsp olive oil
- 1 tsp dried oregano
- 1 tsp garlic powder
- Salt and pepper to taste

For the Mint Yogurt Sauce:
- 1 cup plain Greek yogurt
- 2 tbsp chopped fresh mint
- 1 tbsp lemon juice
- 1 tsp honey
- 1 garlic clove, minced
- Salt and pepper to taste

PROCEDURE:

1. Preheat your grill or grill pan to medium-high heat.

2. In a small bowl, combine the olive oil, oregano, garlic powder, salt, and pepper. Rub this mixture all over the lamb chops.

3. Grill the lamb chops for 3-4 minutes per side, or until they reach your desired doneness. Transfer to a plate and let rest for 5 minutes.

For the Mint Yogurt Sauce:
1. In a small bowl, mix together the Greek yogurt, chopped mint, lemon juice, honey, garlic, salt, and pepper.

2. Serve the grilled lamb chops with the mint yogurt sauce on the side.

This dish is a great option for managing type 2 diabetes for a few reasons:

- Lamb is a lean protein that is low in carbs and high in healthy fats.
- The mint yogurt sauce provides a refreshing, flavorful topping without added sugars.
- Grilling the lamb chops keeps the dish light and healthy.
- Pairing the lamb with a side salad or roasted vegetables makes for a well-balanced, diabetes-friendly meal.

Remember to watch your portion sizes - aim for 3-4 oz of lamb per serving. Enjoy!

102. Herb-Crusted Tilapia

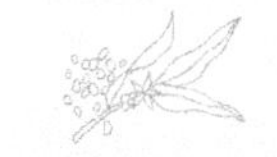

PREP TIME
20 MINUTES

COOK TIME
30 MINUTES

INGREDIENTS:

- 4 (6 oz) tilapia fillets
- 1/4 cup whole wheat breadcrumbs
- 2 tbsp grated Parmesan cheese
- 1 tbsp chopped fresh parsley
- 1 tsp dried oregano
- 1 tsp garlic powder
- 1 tbsp olive oil
- Salt and pepper to taste

PROCEDURE:

1. Preheat your oven to 400°F. Lightly grease a baking sheet or oven-safe dish.

2. In a shallow bowl, combine the breadcrumbs, Parmesan cheese, parsley, oregano, and garlic powder. Season with salt and pepper.

3. Brush the tilapia fillets lightly with the olive oil on both sides.

4. Dredge the tilapia fillets in the breadcrumb mixture, pressing gently to help the coating adhere.

5. Arrange the coated tilapia fillets on the prepared baking sheet.

6. Bake for 12-15 minutes, or until the fish flakes easily with a fork and the coating is golden brown.

7. Serve the herb-crusted tilapia immediately.

This recipe for herb-crusted tilapia is a great option for managing type 2 diabetes for the following reasons:

- Tilapia is a lean, low-mercury fish that is high in protein and low in carbs.
- The whole wheat breadcrumb and Parmesan cheese coating provides a crunchy texture without the need for frying.
- The herbs and spices (parsley, oregano, garlic powder) add flavor without added sugars or high-sodium sauces.
- Baking the tilapia keeps the dish light and healthy.
- Portion control is important, so aim for a 4-6 oz serving of the herb-crusted tilapia.

103. Zucchini Noodles with Pesto and Chicken

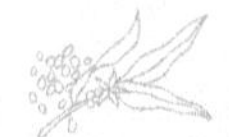

PREP TIME
20 MINUTES

COOK TIME
30 MINUTES

INGREDIENTS :

- 3 medium zucchini, spiralized or julienned into noodles
- 1 lb boneless, skinless chicken breasts, grilled and sliced
- 1/2 cup basil pesto (store-bought or homemade)
- 2 tbsp toasted pine nuts
- 2 tbsp grated Parmesan cheese
- Salt and pepper to taste

PROCEDURE :

1. If using grilled chicken, cook the chicken breasts and slice them into strips. Set aside.

2. In a large skillet or wok, heat the zucchini noodles over medium heat for 2-3 minutes, just until they start to soften slightly. Be careful not to overcook them.

3. Remove the zucchini noodles from the heat and transfer them to a large bowl.

4. Add the sliced grilled chicken and the basil pesto to the bowl. Toss everything together until the noodles and chicken are evenly coated with the pesto.

5. Top the zucchini noodles and chicken with the toasted pine nuts and grated Parmesan cheese.

6. Season with salt and pepper to taste.

7. Serve the zucchini noodles and chicken immediately.

This dish is a great option for managing type 2 diabetes for the following reasons:

- Zucchini noodles are a low-carb, high-fiber alternative to traditional pasta.
- Grilled chicken is a lean protein that is low in carbs and high in protein.
- Basil pesto provides flavor without the need for high-sodium sauces or added sugars.
- The pine nuts and Parmesan cheese add healthy fats to the dish.
- The overall dish is low in carbs and high in fiber, protein, and healthy fats, which can help regulate blood sugar levels.

104. BBQ Chicken with Sweet Potato Fries

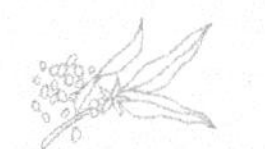

PREP TIME
20 MINUTES

COOK TIME
30 MINUTES

INGREDIENTS:

For the Sweet Potato Fries:
- 2 lbs sweet potatoes, peeled and cut into 1/2-inch thick fries
- 1 tbsp olive oil
- 1 tsp paprika
- 1/2 tsp garlic powder
- Salt and pepper to taste

For the BBQ Chicken:
- 4 boneless, skinless chicken breasts
- 1/2 cup no-sugar-added BBQ sauce
- 1 tsp smoked paprika
- 1/2 tsp garlic powder
- Salt and pepper to taste

PROCEDURE:

1. Preheat your oven to 400°F. Line two baking sheets with parchment paper.

For the Sweet Potato Fries:
1. In a large bowl, toss the sweet potato fries with the olive oil, paprika, garlic powder, salt, and pepper until evenly coated.
2. Spread the fries in a single layer on one of the prepared baking sheets.
3. Bake for 20-25 minutes, flipping halfway, until the fries are tender and lightly browned.

For the BBQ Chicken:
1. In a small bowl, mix together the BBQ sauce, smoked paprika, garlic powder, salt, and pepper.
2. Place the chicken breasts on the second prepared baking sheet and brush them evenly with the BBQ sauce mixture.
3. Bake the chicken for 20-25 minutes, or until it reaches an internal temperature of 165°F.

Serve the BBQ chicken with the roasted sweet potato fries.

This dish is diabetes-friendly for the following reasons:

- Sweet potatoes are a complex carbohydrate that is high in fiber, vitamins, and minerals.
- Boneless, skinless chicken breasts are a lean protein that is low in carbs.
- The no-sugar-added BBQ sauce provides flavor without added sugars.
- Baking the sweet potato fries and chicken keeps the dish light and healthy.
- The combination of protein, complex carbs, and fiber helps regulate blood sugar levels.

105. Vegetable Lasagna with Zucchini Noodles

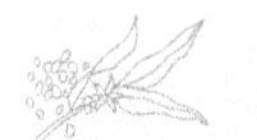 

PREP TIME
20 MINUTES

COOK TIME
30 MINUTES

INGREDIENTS :

- 3 medium zucchini, sliced lengthwise into thin noodle-like strips
- 1 tbsp olive oil
- 1 onion, diced
- 3 cloves garlic, minced
- 8 oz sliced mushrooms
- 1 red bell pepper, diced
- 1 cup baby spinach, chopped
- 1 (15 oz) can no-sugar-added tomato sauce
- 1 tsp dried oregano
- 1/2 tsp dried basil
- Salt and pepper to taste
- 1 cup part-skim ricotta cheese
- 1 cup shredded part-skim mozzarella cheese

PROCEDURE :

1. Preheat your oven to 375°F. Lightly grease a 9x13 inch baking dish.

2. In a large skillet, heat the olive oil over medium heat. Add the onion and garlic and sauté for 2-3 minutes until fragrant.

3. Add the sliced mushrooms and bell pepper to the skillet. Cook for 5-7 minutes, until the vegetables are tender.

4. Stir in the chopped spinach and cook for an additional 2 minutes until wilted. Add the tomato sauce, oregano, basil, salt, and pepper. Simmer for 5 minutes.

5. Spread a thin layer of the vegetable sauce in the bottom of the prepared baking dish.

6. Arrange a layer of the zucchini noodles over the sauce. Top with dollops of the ricotta cheese and a sprinkle of the mozzarella cheese.

7. Repeat the layers of zucchini noodles, vegetable sauce, ricotta, and mozzarella until all the ingredients are used up, ending with the mozzarella cheese on top.

8. Bake the lasagna for 30-35 minutes, until the cheese is melted and bubbly. Let the lasagna cool for 5-10 minutes before serving.

This vegetable lasagna with zucchini noodles is a great option for managing type 2 diabetes because:

- Zucchini noodles replace traditional wheat-based lasagna noodles, reducing the carb content.
- The vegetable-based filling is high in fiber, vitamins, and minerals.

106. Grilled Scallops with Asparagus

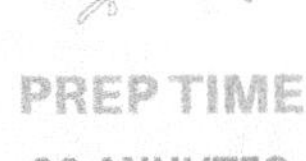 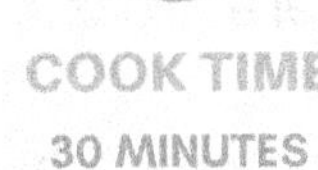

PREP TIME 20 MINUTES | **COOK TIME** 30 MINUTES

INGREDIENTS :

- 1 lb sea scallops, patted dry
- 1 lb asparagus, trimmed
- 2 tbsp olive oil
- 2 tbsp lemon juice
- 1 tsp garlic powder
- 1 tsp dried oregano
- Salt and pepper to taste

PROCEDURE :

1. Preheat grill or grill pan to medium-high heat.

2. In a small bowl, whisk together the olive oil, lemon juice, garlic powder, oregano, salt, and pepper.

3. Thread the scallops onto skewers, leaving a little space between each one.

4. Toss the asparagus spears with 1 tbsp of the lemon-herb mixture.

5. Grill the scallop skewers for 2-3 minutes per side, until opaque and cooked through.

6. Grill the asparagus for 5-7 minutes, turning occasionally, until tender-crisp.

7. Serve the grilled scallops and asparagus immediately, drizzling any remaining lemon-herb mixture over the top.

This recipe is diabetes-friendly for the following reasons:

- Scallops are a lean, high-protein seafood that is low in carbs.
- Asparagus is a non-starchy vegetable that is high in fiber, vitamins, and minerals.
- The lemon and herb seasoning adds flavor without the need for added sugars or high-sodium sauces.
- Grilling the scallops and asparagus keeps the dish light and healthy.

Portion control is still important, so aim for 4-6 scallops and 1 cup of asparagus per serving. This dish pairs well with a side salad or a small serving of whole grains like quinoa or brown rice.

107. Roasted Turkey Breast with Vegetables

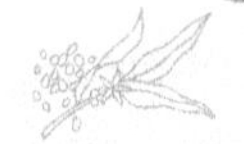

PREP TIME
20 MINUTES

COOK TIME
30 MINUTES

INGREDIENTS :

- 1 (3-4 lb) bone-in, skin-on turkey breast
- 2 tbsp olive oil
- 1 tsp dried thyme
- 1 tsp garlic powder
- 1/2 tsp salt
- 1/4 tsp black pepper
- 2 cups cubed butternut squash
- 2 cups Brussels sprouts, trimmed and halved
- 1 red onion, cut into wedges
- 2 cloves garlic, minced

PROCEDURE :

1. Preheat your oven to 375°F. Lightly grease a large roasting pan or baking sheet.

2. Pat the turkey breast dry with paper towels and place it in the prepared roasting pan.

3. In a small bowl, mix together the olive oil, thyme, garlic powder, salt, and pepper. Rub this seasoning mixture all over the turkey breast.

4. Arrange the cubed butternut squash, Brussels sprouts, red onion wedges, and minced garlic around the turkey breast in the roasting pan.

5. Roast the turkey and vegetables for 1 to 1 1/2 hours, or until the turkey reaches an internal temperature of 165°F. Baste the turkey occasionally with the pan juices.

6. Let the turkey rest for 10-15 minutes before slicing and serving. Serve the roasted turkey breast with the roasted vegetables.

This roasted turkey breast with vegetables dish is a great option for managing type 2 diabetes for the following reasons:

- Turkey breast is a lean protein that is low in carbs and high in protein.
- Butternut squash and Brussels sprouts are non-starchy vegetables that are high in fiber, vitamins, and minerals.
- The simple seasoning of thyme, garlic, salt, and pepper adds flavor without the need for high-sodium sauces or added sugars.
- Roasting the turkey and vegetables keeps the dish light and healthy.
- The combination of protein, fiber, and complex carbs helps regulate blood sugar levels.

108. Stuffed Cabbage Rolls

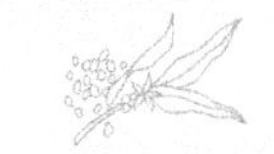 

PREP TIME
20 MINUTES

COOK TIME
30 MINUTES

INGREDIENTS :

- 1 medium head green cabbage
- 1 lb ground turkey
- 1 cup cooked brown rice
- 1 onion, finely chopped
- 2 cloves garlic, minced
- 1 tsp dried oregano
- 1/2 tsp dried thyme
- 1/4 tsp red pepper flakes (optional)
- Salt and pepper to taste
- 1 (15 oz) can no-sugar-added tomato sauce
- 1/4 cup low-sodium chicken or vegetable broth

PROCEDURE :

1. Bring a large pot of water to a boil. Core the cabbage and carefully place it in the boiling water. Cook for 3-5 minutes, until the outer leaves are softened. Remove the cabbage leaves one by one as they become pliable.

2. In a large bowl, combine the ground turkey, cooked brown rice, onion, garlic, oregano, thyme, red pepper flakes (if using), salt, and pepper. Mix well.

3. Place about 1/4 cup of the turkey mixture onto the center of each cabbage leaf. Fold the sides of the leaf over the filling and then roll up tightly.

4. Arrange the stuffed cabbage rolls seam-side down in a large baking dish. Pour the tomato sauce and chicken/vegetable broth over the top.

5. Cover the baking dish with foil and bake at 375°F for 45-60 minutes, until the cabbage is tender and the filling is cooked through. Serve the stuffed cabbage rolls warm.

This stuffed cabbage roll recipe is a great option for managing type 2 diabetes for the following reasons:

- Cabbage is a low-carb, high-fiber vegetable that serves as the "wrapper" for the filling.
- Ground turkey is a lean protein that is low in carbs and high in protein.
- Brown rice provides complex carbohydrates and fiber.
- The tomato sauce provides flavor without added sugars.
- Baking the stuffed cabbage rolls keeps the dish light and healthy.

109. Baked Trout with Almonds

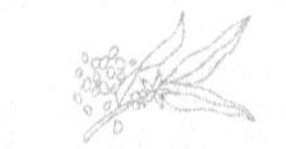

PREP TIME
20 MINUTES

COOK TIME
30 MINUTES

INGREDIENTS :

- 4 (6 oz) trout fillets
- 2 tbsp olive oil
- 1/4 cup sliced almonds
- 1 tsp lemon zest
- 1 tbsp lemon juice
- 1 tsp dried parsley
- 1/4 tsp garlic powder
- Salt and pepper to taste

PROCEDURE :

1. Preheat your oven to 400°F. Lightly grease a baking sheet or oven-safe dish.

2. Place the trout fillets skin-side down on the prepared baking sheet.

3. In a small bowl, mix together the olive oil, sliced almonds, lemon zest, lemon juice, dried parsley, garlic powder, salt, and pepper.

4. Spoon the almond mixture evenly over the top of the trout fillets, pressing it gently to help it adhere.

5. Bake the trout for 12-15 minutes, or until it flakes easily with a fork and reaches an internal temperature of 145°F.

6. Serve the baked trout with almonds immediately.

This recipe for baked trout with almonds is a great option for managing type 2 diabetes for the following reasons:

- Trout is a lean, high-protein fish that is low in carbs and high in healthy omega-3 fatty acids.
- Almonds provide a crunchy, flavorful topping that is rich in healthy fats and fiber.
- The lemon, parsley, and garlic add flavor without the need for high-sodium sauces or added sugars.
- Baking the trout keeps the dish light and healthy.
- The combination of protein, healthy fats, and minimal carbs helps regulate blood sugar levels.

Portion control is still important, so aim for a 4-6 oz serving of the baked trout per person. Serve with a side of roasted vegetables or a fresh salad for a complete, diabetes-friendly meal.

110. Chicken Marsala with Cauliflower Mash

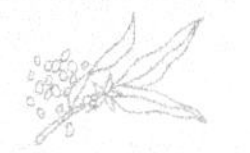 

PREP TIME	COOK TIME
20 MINUTES	30 MINUTES

INGREDIENTS:

For the Chicken Marsala:
- 4 (6 oz) boneless, skinless chicken breasts
- 2 tbsp olive oil
- 8 oz sliced mushrooms
- 1/2 cup Marsala wine
- 1/2 cup low-sodium chicken broth
- 2 tbsp unsalted butter
- 1 tsp dried thyme
- Salt and pepper to taste

For the Cauliflower Mash:
- 1 head of cauliflower, cut into florets
- 2 tbsp unsalted butter
- 1/4 cup unsweetened almond milk
- 1/4 cup grated Parmesan cheese
- 1 tsp garlic powder
- Salt and pepper to taste

PROCEDURE:

1. Preheat your oven to 400°F.

For the Chicken Marsala:
1. Season the chicken breasts with salt and pepper.
2. Heat the olive oil in a large skillet over medium-high heat. Add the chicken and cook for 3-4 minutes per side until browned.
3. Transfer the chicken to a baking sheet and bake for 12-15 minutes, until cooked through.
4. In the same skillet, sauté the mushrooms for 3-4 minutes until tender.
5. Add the Marsala wine, chicken broth, butter, and thyme. Simmer for 5-7 minutes until the sauce has thickened slightly.
6. Return the cooked chicken to the skillet and coat with the Marsala sauce.

For the Cauliflower Mash:
1. Steam the cauliflower florets until very tender, about 10-12 minutes.
2. Drain the cauliflower and transfer to a food processor. Add the butter, almond milk, Parmesan, garlic powder, salt, and pepper.
3. Pulse the mixture until smooth and creamy.

Serve the chicken Marsala over the cauliflower mash.

This dish is diabetes-friendly for the following reasons:

- Chicken is a lean protein that is low in carbs.
- Cauliflower is a low-carb, high-fiber vegetable that replaces traditional mashed potatoes.
- The Marsala wine and mushrooms add flavor without the need for high-sodium sauces.
- Portion control is important, so aim for a 4-6 oz serving of chicken and 1/2 cup of cauliflower mash.

111. Roasted Brussels Sprouts

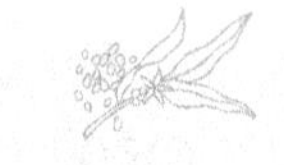

PREP TIME
20 MINUTES

COOK TIME
30 MINUTES

INGREDIENTS:

- 1 lb Brussels sprouts, trimmed and halved
- 2 tbsp olive oil
- 1 tsp garlic powder
- 1/2 tsp dried thyme
- 1/4 tsp red pepper flakes (optional)
- Salt and pepper to taste

PROCEDURE:

1. Preheat your oven to 400°F. Line a baking sheet with parchment paper.

2. In a large bowl, toss the trimmed and halved Brussels sprouts with the olive oil, garlic powder, dried thyme, red pepper flakes (if using), salt, and pepper.

3. Spread the Brussels sprouts in a single layer on the prepared baking sheet.

4. Roast the Brussels sprouts for 20-25 minutes, tossing halfway through, until they are tender and lightly browned.

5. Serve the roasted Brussels sprouts immediately.

This recipe for roasted Brussels sprouts is a great option for managing type 2 diabetes for the following reasons:

- Brussels sprouts are a non-starchy, fiber-rich vegetable that is low in carbs.
- The simple seasoning of garlic powder, thyme, and optional red pepper flakes adds flavor without the need for added sugars or high-sodium sauces.
- Roasting the Brussels sprouts brings out their natural sweetness and creates a crispy texture.
- Portion control is important, so aim for a 1/2 cup serving of the roasted Brussels sprouts.

Roasted Brussels sprouts make a great side dish to grilled or baked protein, such as chicken, fish, or tofu. You can also toss them with a small serving of whole grains, like quinoa or brown rice, for a more substantial meal.

112. Cauliflower Mash

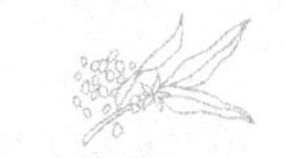 

PREP TIME
20 MINUTES

COOK TIME
30 MINUTES

INGREDIENTS:

- 1 large head of cauliflower, cut into florets
- 2 tbsp unsalted butter
- 1/4 cup unsweetened almond milk
- 2 tbsp grated Parmesan cheese
- 1 tsp garlic powder
- 1/2 tsp dried thyme
- Salt and pepper to taste

PROCEDURE:

1. In a large pot, bring 1-2 inches of water to a boil. Add the cauliflower florets, cover, and steam for 10-12 minutes, until very tender.

2. Drain the cooked cauliflower and transfer it to a food processor or high-powered blender.

3. Add the butter, almond milk, Parmesan cheese, garlic powder, and dried thyme to the food processor.

4. Blend the ingredients together until the cauliflower is smooth and creamy, scraping down the sides as needed.

5. Season the cauliflower mash with salt and pepper to taste. Serve the cauliflower mash warm.

This cauliflower mash is a great option for managing type 2 diabetes for the following reasons:

- Cauliflower is a low-carb, high-fiber vegetable that serves as a healthier alternative to traditional mashed potatoes.
- The small amount of butter and Parmesan cheese provides healthy fats without added sugars.
- The almond milk adds creaminess without the carbs found in regular dairy milk.
- The garlic and thyme seasoning adds flavor without the need for high-sodium sauces.

Portion control is still important, so aim for a 1/2 cup serving of the cauliflower mash. This dish makes a great side to grilled or roasted protein, such as chicken, fish, or pork.

The combination of low-carb, high-fiber vegetables and healthy fats can help regulate blood sugar levels for those managing type 2 diabetes.

113. Sautéed Spinach with Garlic

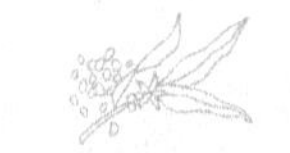

PREP TIME
20 MINUTES

COOK TIME
30 MINUTES

INGREDIENTS :

- 1 lb fresh spinach, washed and stems removed
- 1 tbsp olive oil
- 3 cloves garlic, minced
- 1/4 tsp red pepper flakes (optional)
- Salt and pepper to taste

PROCEDURE :

1. In a large skillet or wok, heat the olive oil over medium heat.

2. Add the minced garlic and red pepper flakes (if using) to the hot oil. Sauté for 1-2 minutes, until fragrant.

3. Add the fresh spinach to the skillet in batches, stirring constantly, until the spinach is wilted down and tender, about 3-5 minutes total.

4. Season the sautéed spinach with salt and pepper to taste.

5. Serve the sautéed spinach with garlic immediately.

This sautéed spinach dish is a great option for managing type 2 diabetes for the following reasons:

- Spinach is a non-starchy, nutrient-dense vegetable that is low in carbs and high in fiber, vitamins, and minerals.
- The small amount of olive oil provides healthy fats without adding significant carbs.
- The garlic and optional red pepper flakes add flavor without the need for high-sodium sauces or added sugars.
- Sautéing the spinach quickly preserves its nutrients and texture.

Portion control is still important, so aim for a 1/2 to 1 cup serving of the sautéed spinach. This dish makes a great side to grilled or baked protein, such as chicken, fish, or tofu. It can also be incorporated into other dishes, like omelets or salads, for an extra boost of nutrients.

114. Quinoa Pilaf

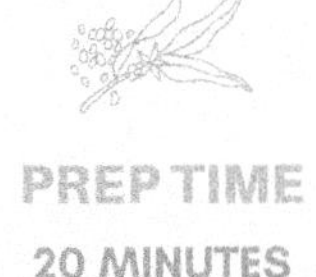

PREP TIME
20 MINUTES

COOK TIME
30 MINUTES

INGREDIENTS:

- 1 cup uncooked quinoa, rinsed
- 2 cups low-sodium chicken or vegetable broth
- 1 tbsp olive oil
- 1 onion, diced
- 2 cloves garlic, minced
- 1 cup diced bell peppers (any color)
- 1 cup diced zucchini
- 1/4 cup chopped fresh parsley
- 1 tsp dried thyme
- Salt and pepper to taste

PROCEDURE:

1. In a medium saucepan, combine the rinsed quinoa and broth. Bring to a boil, then reduce heat to low, cover, and simmer for 15-20 minutes, until the quinoa is tender and the liquid is absorbed.

2. While the quinoa is cooking, heat the olive oil in a large skillet over medium heat. Add the diced onion and sauté for 3-4 minutes until translucent.

3. Add the minced garlic, diced bell peppers, and diced zucchini to the skillet. Sauté for an additional 5-7 minutes, until the vegetables are tender-crisp.

4. Fluff the cooked quinoa with a fork and transfer it to the skillet with the sautéed vegetables.

5. Stir in the chopped parsley and dried thyme. Season with salt and pepper to taste. Serve the quinoa pilaf warm.

This quinoa pilaf is a great option for managing type 2 diabetes for the following reasons:

- Quinoa is a high-fiber, high-protein grain that is low in the glycemic index.
- The vegetables (bell peppers, zucchini) provide fiber, vitamins, and minerals without adding a significant amount of carbs.
- The simple seasoning of parsley and thyme adds flavor without the need for high-sodium sauces or added sugars.
- The overall dish is balanced with complex carbs, protein, and fiber to help regulate blood sugar levels.

Portion control is still important, so aim for a 3/4 to 1 cup serving of the quinoa pilaf. This dish can be served as a main course or as a side to grilled or roasted protein.

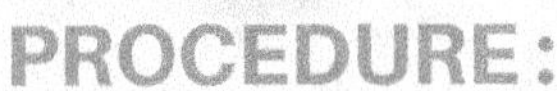
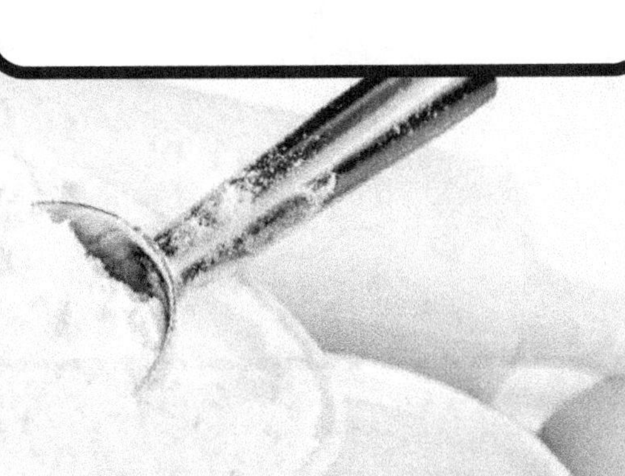

115. Green Bean Almondine

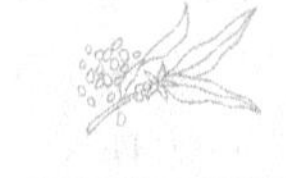

PREP TIME
20 MINUTES

COOK TIME
30 MINUTES

INGREDIENTS:

- 1 lb fresh green beans, trimmed
- 2 tbsp unsalted butter
- 1/4 cup sliced almonds
- 1 tbsp lemon juice
- Salt and pepper to taste

PROCEDURE:

1. Bring a large pot of salted water to a boil. Add the green beans and cook for 3-5 minutes until tender-crisp. Drain and rinse with cold water to stop the cooking.

2. In a skillet, melt the butter over medium heat. Add the sliced almonds and cook, stirring frequently, until the almonds are lightly toasted, about 2-3 minutes.

3. Add the cooked green beans to the skillet with the toasted almonds. Toss to coat the beans in the butter and almonds.

4. Drizzle the lemon juice over the green bean almondine and season with salt and pepper to taste.

5. Serve the green bean almondine warm. Enjoy!

The key elements are the toasted almonds, lemon juice, and simple preparation to let the fresh green bean flavor shine. This makes a great side dish to complement many main courses.

116. Cucumber and Tomato Salad

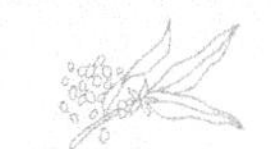 

PREP TIME
20 MINUTES

COOK TIME
30 MINUTES

INGREDIENTS :

- 2 medium cucumbers, sliced
- 2 cups cherry or grape tomatoes, halved
- 1/2 red onion, thinly sliced
- 2 tbsp red wine vinegar
- 1 tbsp olive oil
- 1 tsp dried oregano
- 1/4 tsp salt
- 1/4 tsp black pepper
- 2 tbsp chopped fresh basil (optional)

PROCEDURE :

1. In a large bowl, combine the sliced cucumbers, halved tomatoes, and thinly sliced red onion.

2. In a small bowl, whisk together the red wine vinegar, olive oil, dried oregano, salt, and black pepper.

3. Pour the vinaigrette over the cucumber and tomato mixture and toss gently to coat.

4. If desired, sprinkle the chopped fresh basil over the top of the salad.

5. Refrigerate the salad for at least 30 minutes to allow the flavors to meld.

6. Serve the cucumber and tomato salad chilled.

This cucumber and tomato salad is a great option for managing type 2 diabetes for the following reasons:

- Cucumbers and tomatoes are non-starchy, fiber-rich vegetables that are low in carbs.
- The red wine vinegar and olive oil provide a flavorful, low-calorie dressing without added sugars.
- The fresh herbs (oregano, basil) add flavor without the need for high-sodium sauces.
- The overall dish is low in calories and carbs, making it a diabetes-friendly choice.

Portion control is still important, so aim for a 1-cup serving of the salad. This dish makes a great side to grilled or baked protein, or it can be enjoyed on its own as a refreshing and healthy snack.

The combination of fiber, vitamins, and minimal carbs in this cucumber and tomato salad makes it a great option for managing type 2 diabetes.

117. Grilled Asparagus

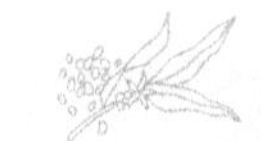 

PREP TIME
20 MINUTES

COOK TIME
30 MINUTES

INGREDIENTS:

- 1 lb asparagus, trimmed
- 1 tbsp olive oil
- 1 tsp lemon zest
- 1 tsp lemon juice
- 1/2 tsp garlic powder
- 1/4 tsp salt
- 1/4 tsp black pepper

PROCEDURE:

1. Preheat your grill or grill pan to medium-high heat.

2. In a large bowl, toss the trimmed asparagus spears with the olive oil, lemon zest, lemon juice, garlic powder, salt, and pepper until the asparagus is evenly coated.

3. Arrange the seasoned asparagus in a single layer on the preheated grill or grill pan.

4. Grill the asparagus for 5-7 minutes, turning occasionally, until tender-crisp and slightly charred.

5. Serve the grilled asparagus immediately.

This grilled asparagus recipe is a great option for managing type 2 diabetes for the following reasons:

- Asparagus is a non-starchy, fiber-rich vegetable that is low in carbs.
- The simple seasoning of lemon, garlic, salt, and pepper adds flavor without the need for high-sodium sauces or added sugars.
- Grilling the asparagus adds a delicious, smoky flavor while keeping the dish light and healthy.
- Asparagus is a good source of vitamins, minerals, and antioxidants that can be beneficial for managing diabetes.

Portion control is still important, so aim for a 1/2 to 1 cup serving of the grilled asparagus. This dish makes a great side to grilled or baked protein, such as chicken, fish, or tofu. You can also toss the grilled asparagus with a small serving of whole grains, like quinoa or brown rice, for a more substantial meal.

118. Sweet Potato Wedges

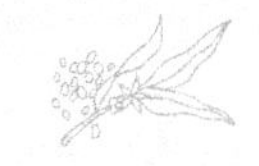

PREP TIME
20 MINUTES

COOK TIME
30 MINUTES

INGREDIENTS:

- 2 lbs sweet potatoes, washed and cut into 1/2-inch thick wedges
- 2 tbsp olive oil
- 1 tsp paprika
- 1 tsp garlic powder
- 1/2 tsp ground cumin
- 1/4 tsp cayenne pepper (optional)
- Salt and pepper to taste

PROCEDURE:

1. Preheat your oven to 400°F. Line a large baking sheet with parchment paper.

2. In a large bowl, toss the sweet potato wedges with the olive oil, paprika, garlic powder, cumin, and cayenne pepper (if using). Season with salt and pepper.

3. Arrange the seasoned sweet potato wedges in a single layer on the prepared baking sheet, making sure they are not overcrowded.

4. Bake for 20-25 minutes, flipping the wedges halfway through, until they are tender and lightly browned.

5. Serve the sweet potato wedges immediately.

This recipe for sweet potato wedges is a great option for managing type 2 diabetes for the following reasons:

- Sweet potatoes are a complex carbohydrate that is high in fiber, vitamins, and minerals. They have a lower glycemic index compared to regular potatoes, which helps regulate blood sugar levels.
- The spices and seasonings (paprika, garlic powder, cumin, cayenne) add flavor without the need for added sugars or high-sodium sauces.
- Baking the sweet potato wedges instead of frying them reduces the amount of fat and calories.
- Portion control is important, so aim for a 1/2 cup serving of the sweet potato wedges.

These sweet potato wedges can be enjoyed as a side dish or as a healthy snack. Pair them with grilled or roasted protein, such as chicken or fish, and a side salad for a complete, diabetes-friendly meal.

119. Broccoli and Cheese Bake

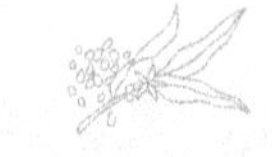

PREP TIME
20 MINUTES

COOK TIME
30 MINUTES

INGREDIENTS :

- 1 lb broccoli florets, cut into bite-sized pieces
- 2 tbsp unsalted butter
- 2 tbsp all-purpose flour
- 1 cup milk
- 1 cup shredded cheddar cheese
- 1/4 cup grated Parmesan cheese
- 1/4 tsp garlic powder
- Salt and pepper to taste
- 1/2 cup breadcrumbs or crushed crackers

PROCEDURE :

1. Preheat the oven to 375°F. Grease a 9x13 inch baking dish.

2. Bring a large pot of salted water to a boil. Add the broccoli florets and cook for 3-5 minutes until tender-crisp. Drain and set aside.

3. In a saucepan, melt the butter over medium heat. Whisk in the flour and cook for 1 minute. Gradually whisk in the milk and cook until thickened, about 5 minutes.

4. Remove the sauce from heat and stir in the cheddar cheese, Parmesan cheese, garlic powder, salt, and pepper until the cheese is melted and the sauce is smooth.

5. Add the cooked broccoli to the cheese sauce and stir to coat. Transfer the mixture to the prepared baking dish.

6. Sprinkle the breadcrumbs or crushed crackers evenly over the top.

7. Bake for 20-25 minutes, until the topping is golden brown and the sauce is bubbly.

8. Let stand for 5 minutes before serving.

Enjoy this creamy, cheesy broccoli bake as a delicious side dish! The breadcrumb topping adds a nice crunch.

120. Zucchini Noodles with Pesto

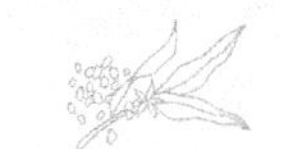 

PREP TIME
20 MINUTES

COOK TIME
30 MINUTES

INGREDIENTS :

- 3-4 medium zucchinis, spiralized or julienned into noodles
- 1/2 cup basil pesto (store-bought or homemade)
- 1/4 cup cherry tomatoes, halved
- 2 tbsp toasted pine nuts
- 2 tbsp grated Parmesan cheese
- Salt and pepper to taste

PROCEDURE :

1. If using whole zucchinis, spiralize or julienne them into long, thin noodle-like strips.

2. In a large bowl, toss the zucchini noodles with the basil pesto until the noodles are evenly coated.

3. Add the halved cherry tomatoes, toasted pine nuts, and grated Parmesan cheese. Toss gently to combine.

4. Season with salt and pepper to taste.

5. Serve the zucchini noodles with pesto immediately, while the noodles are still crisp.

Optional Variations:

- Top with grilled or sautéed chicken or shrimp for a protein-packed meal.

- Add a sprinkle of red pepper flakes for a little heat.

- Substitute the basil pesto with another type of pesto, like sun-dried tomato or arugula pesto.

- Garnish with fresh basil leaves or chopped parsley.

The zucchini noodles provide a low-carb, veggie-based alternative to traditional pasta, while the pesto, tomatoes, and nuts add tons of flavor and texture. Enjoy this fresh and healthy dish!

As you conclude your journey through the **"Type 2 Diabetes Cookbook for 1 Person: 110+ Quick and Healthy Recipes for Busy Individuals with Type 2 Diabetes,"** we hope you've discovered a wealth of delicious, practical solutions for managing your diabetes with ease and enjoyment.

This cookbook was crafted with the understanding that busy schedules and solo dining should not stand in the way of healthy eating. Each of the over 110 recipes included in this book has been thoughtfully designed to offer quick, nutritious meals that support stable blood sugar levels without sacrificing taste or convenience.

Beyond recipes, you've found valuable tips on portion control, ingredient selection, and efficient meal planning strategies tailored specifically for individuals managing Type 2 diabetes alone. These insights are intended to empower you to make informed choices that contribute to your overall health and well-being.

We encourage you to continue exploring new flavors, experimenting with ingredients, and discovering the pleasure of preparing meals that nourish both body and soul. With this cookbook as your guide, managing diabetes can be not just manageable, but a source of culinary inspiration and satisfaction.

Thank you for choosing this cookbook to support your journey toward healthier eating habits. Here's to balanced blood sugar, delicious meals enjoyed solo, and a future filled with culinary delight and good health. Cheers to you and your well-being!